GETTING FIT
The
Hard
Way

GETTING FIT
The Hard Way

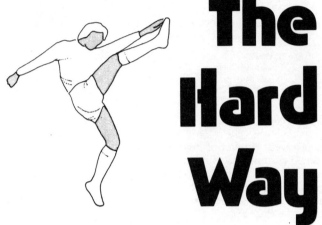

Barry Walsh & Peter Douglas

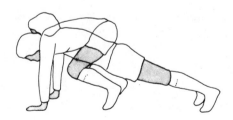

BLANDFORD PRESS
Poole   Dorset

First published in the U.K. 1981 by Blandford Press Ltd,
Link House, West Street,
Poole, Dorset BH15 1LL
Copyright © 1981 Barry Walsh and Peter Douglas

British Library Cataloguing in Publication Data

Walsh, Barry
    Getting fit, the hard way.
    1. Exercise   2. Physical fitness
    I. Title
    613.7'1   RA781

ISBN 07137 1086 1

Typeset in 11/12pt Plantin and 9/10 Univers, printed
and bound in England by Staples Printers Rochester Ltd
at the Stanhope Press

*Dedicated to all those who 'haven't got the time to exercise',
for they are in most need of this book.*

Contents

Introduction

Technical innovation during this century has meant that an increasing amount of work formerly performed by muscle power is now done by some form of technical device. Much of this change is for the better, but it leaves us with a problem we have only gone some way towards solving: namely, the possession of a body that was designed for action – and pretty demanding action at that. The physical requirements necessary to get through an average Stone Age day would make almost impossible demands upon us in the 1980s.

In the advanced industrial nations of the world, we now have a considerable wealth of leisure time on our hands and we can look forward to a lot more. However, if we are to keep our bodies in anything like reasonable condition it will be necessary to spend a significant part of this leisure time in physical recreation.

The well-publicised dangers of being unfit have habitually failed to produce the required response from most people. Men and women, it seems, are by nature gamblers, prepared to take the risks that poor physical condition can create. They assume they will prove to be the exception to the rule and will avoid the consequences of a life of inactivity with all its associated problems.

Many of us have assumed that technology and modern thinking can help us to get into shape without the necessary physical effort. People have resorted to many gadgets, theories and specialised diets that promised all kinds of physical benefits. But, unfortunately, getting fit is not just another task that can be performed for us by the right kind of machine.

The fact remains that effort itself is an integral part of getting fit. Hence the title of this book: Getting Fit – The Hard Way. We believe that, with a little commitment from you it is possible to achieve a state of physical wellbeing that will enhance every aspect of your life. Between the covers of this book you will, however, find nothing revolutionary or startlingly original. What you will find is an *honest* manual of exercise with information to tell you 'Why' rather than just 'How' to get fit.

Many people look back to the time, usually at school, when they were really fit and life seemed much more fun; a time when they were probably more attractive and more energetic. Then, physical tasks did not feel onerous and concern about a state of fitness did not occupy the mind. Well, it is possible to attain something like that state of fitness again, but it is *not* going to be easy.

When you get round to selecting the routines in this book that suit you best, think also of taking up a sport that is sensibly within your capabilities. Interest in a sport provides an additional spur to continue with a fitness programme. And once fit you have the right base from which to improve skill and all round ability. However, remember that *appropriate* sport is the key: it is not a good idea to take up rugby in your mid-forties just because you were once a nifty scrum-half in school.

There are also many who do not take part in sport and have no wish to do so. This is fine, for we believe that being fit is an end in itself and a more than adequate answer to the cynical question often posed – Fit for what?

The authors are all too well aware that those who are dedicated to a life of inactivity invariably possess a savage sense of humour that seems at its best when directed at those trying to get into shape. Brand new track suits have been known to shrink following a withering comment from one of these cynics. The best response is to laugh along with them and keep going because every aspiring exerciser put off represents a small victory for these people.

Console and encourage yourself with the knowledge that they are going to need their sense of humour as the years go by and they slowly degenerate, becoming less mobile, gaining weight and generally succumbing to all those ailments that accompany a lack of physical fitness.

So, particularly in the early stages of your fitness programme:

– Ignore the stares of your neighbours as you creep out of the front door in your track suit, trying harder to become invisible than to run.

– Do not be put off by the barely suppressed hysterics of your spouse as you struggle heroically to perform your third press-up on the bedroom floor.

– Pour scorn on the old joke about keeping fit by going to the funerals of those who exercise.

– Close your ears to stories like the one about the young squash player everyone seems to know who dropped dead in the shower at the age of thirty!

Finally, we repeat the advice given by all fitness books and their associated experts and that is to have a medical check-up if you are in any doubt about your physical ability to take up an exercise programme. We offer some additional advice: if you *do not plan* to get fit, become acquainted with your doctor now, for you will be seeing a lot of each other over the coming years.

Getting fit the hard way can also be the enjoyable way. If you want to get fit *there really is no other way.*

How to Use this Book

This book is designed to help you achieve a state of all round fitness. It contains a number of exercises that can be performed by people of almost any age, without necessarily using apparatus of any kind. Most of the exercises can be performed on your own, in or out of doors. Others are designed for work with a partner of roughly the same age and stage of fitness.

All the exercises are *graded* as suitable for the Unfit (* one star rating), Medium Fit (** two star) and the Superfit (*** three star). How you assess your starting grade is discussed in the following chapters, and it is the purpose of this book to help you progress – from whatever starting point – to the Superfit grade.

The book is divided in two sections. One contains a number of exercises, with illustrations and clear descriptions of how they should be performed. The other section is devoted to a number of fitness-related topics, such as heart, circulation, breathing, muscle structure, diets, food, nutrition, relaxation, sleep, ideal height and weight ratio, etc. You should study the narrative section in addition to learning the exercises, in order to understand the whole *purpose* of becoming fitter. The exercise routines are divided into six main groups:

Exercises for Warm-up
Introduction to Strength and Stamina Training
Exercises mainly for Arms and Shoulders
Exercises mainly for the Chest
Exercises mainly for the Stomach and Back
Exercises mainly for the Legs

Exercising one section of the body invariably affects another part and the groupings are intended only to indicate the main emphasis of the particular routine. For example, exercises involving the upper part of the legs improve the muscle tone of the abdomen, although the specific exercise might be classified under 'legs'.

You are frequently reminded of the importance of *warming up* before

9

engaging in any serious exercise. Failure to warm up correctly can result in unnecessary strains and sprains. For those classifying themselves as Unfit, only the warm-up routines should be performed for the first four weeks or so. This will enable the body to loosen up and become accustomed to the extra demands you are going to make upon it.

As you progress to Strength and Stamina exercises, and routines involving weights, you should concentrate at first on performing the correct movement and using a very light weight only. Even warm-up movements should not be performed too vigorously at first, to avoid stretching and tearing muscle tissue.

The warm-up routines are also used by all grades before *any* session using weights or involving Strength and Stamina routines. The gradings then indicate the number of *repetitions* of each movement, and the number of *sets*, e.g. two groups of 10 repetitions.

Once you have passed Unfit there is a fairly easy progression to Medium Fit as early improvement is rapid and more noticeable. There is then a considerable uplift from Medium Fit to Superfit and only when you can comfortably handle the suggested number of repetitions at Medium Fit grade *over a period of time* should you make the jump to Superfit.

Where weights are used suggested poundages are rarely indicated. This is because strength varies considerably between one person and another and it is important that you choose a weight you can *comfortably handle* for the correct number of repetitions rather than attempting to handle poundages you can barely lift. You should study the section of the book dealing with weight *training* before attempting these exercises.

Finally, it is important that all routines – with or without weights – are performed at a fairly brisk pace, with the minimum of rest in between. An exercise session will therefore normally last less than one hour, although sportsmen and others in the Superfit category may spend considerably more time than this.

What is Fitness?

Before embarking upon any programme designed to improve one's personal fitness level, it is useful to understand what is meant by the term *fitness*. Unfortunately, it is not easy to arrive at a precise definition although a number of authorities have attempted to do just that. According to the USA President's Council on Physical Fitness and Sport, fitness is defined as 'the ability to carry out daily tasks efficiently with enough energy left over to enjoy leisure time pursuits and to meet unforeseen emergencies'. Dr Vaughan Thomas produces a similar but simpler definition and describes fitness as 'enough physical capacity to cope with the physical needs of life'. What those *physical needs* are will vary from one person to another. The professional footballer will, for example, require a higher level of personal fitness in order to survive the game than the average non-sportsman who is nonetheless concerned about maintaining a reasonably high level of all-round fitness. Fitness and health are not the same thing: you may be healthy (i.e. you are not actually ill) but unable to sprint, lift a weight or swim one length of the pool.

Fitness is also personal and specific to the individual, and made up of a number of components, including the following:

Strength
The ability of the muscles to perform work, such as lift a weight or ride a bicycle.

Endurance
Allied to strength, but includes the ability to perform a specific task for a number of repetitions, e.g. to do a hundred press-ups.

Flexibility or suppleness
The ability to perform a wide range of body movements without causing undue strain.

11

Speed
The ability to perform movements quickly and to react quickly, e.g. to catch a cricket ball.

Stamina
The ability to keep going, e.g. during a 90 minute game of soccer, without undue tiring.

CR Fitness
Cardio-vascular (heart and circulation) and respiratory (lungs and breathing) fitness. The ability of the heart and lungs to perform efficiently and at high level when required, and to recover quickly after exertion.

Other components
Fitness also involves agility, co-ordination, balance and dexterity – factors that are particularly important for the sportsman. But the foundation of any fitness programme is CR fitness, linked to increased muscular strength and endurance, and an improvement in stamina, sometimes known as core endurance and linked inevitably to strength.

An improvement in fitness level invariably leads to a feeling of 'well-being' that is not just an absence of illness, but is the ability to perform more effectively in every area of life. Some experts describe this feeling as a 'high', a real sense of exhilaration, enabling them to seemingly sail through life and cope effectively with work, leisure and every other aspect of life with consummate ease. Whereas specific fitness will prepare you for the special demands of individual sports – the stamina of the racing cyclist, the strength of the oarsman, the balance and flexibility of the gymnast, here exercise involves training the body (or parts of it) to perform specific movements with increasing dexterity.

An important element in improved fitness is the degree to which extra stress can be put upon the body, when required, and its ability to recover and return to normal within a comparatively short space of time. Improved CR fitness will result in a lower resting pulse rate, a more powerful heart and more efficient circulation, and the ability to use the lungs to their full capacity to bring oxygen to the muscles and avoid fatigue and cramp. These aspects are examined more fully in later sections.

'Fitness for life' involves improving personal levels of fitness, in line with demands placed on the body, with the result that the body moves into a higher gear, operates at a more efficient level, and has capacity to spare.

How Fit are You?

Before attempting any exercise programme you must determine your own personal state of fitness, in order to decide at which level you should begin and the level that you wish to attain. The young person, fresh from school, who has regularly taken part in games and gymnastics, is likely to be in a better state of fitness than the older man or woman who has taken on the responsibilities of work and marriage and has perhaps neglected to exercise for a number of years. For them progress will be harder, but fortunately it is almost never too late to begin.

If you are in any doubt about your state of health you should consult your doctor and, if necessary, undergo a thorough physical examination, and only start on an exercise programme when you have your doctor's approval. In virtually every case the doctor will be the first one to applaud your decision to get fitter.

There are a number of contributory causes to our general state of unfitness, many of them the so-called diseases of civilisation. These include inactivity, overweight, stress, and destructive habits such as smoking and excessive alcohol consumption. As a result the unfit person is fairly easy to recognise. He can be of any age and is likely to be overweight. Excess weight inhibits activity, and a vicious circle is set up.

Rushed meals, taken at your desk or in the bar, result in an unbalanced diet, the consequences of which include chronic indigestion, flatulence, constipation and other ailments caused by starchy, processed foods.

A feeling of tiredness in the evenings and general lassitude are further common symptoms, while physical exhaustion after even moderate activity, stiffness and aching muscles, are signs that you are out of condition. Sleeplessness and nervous habits also indicate that the body is not being given sufficient physical work.

Walking to the station, the occasional round of golf or even the weekly squash game are not by themselves sufficiently vigorous exercises to make any serious demands on the heart and lungs to produce a state of all-round fitness. Even those who engage in manual work or train with weights to develop their physique may not necessarily be fit. Muscular development may be uneven and circulation and lung capacity seriously under par.

Smokers should very seriously consider giving up the habit. Smoking is a debilitating factor, causing proven damage to the lungs, reducing appetite and causing strain on the heart.

It is essential then to take personal stock of yourself. If you are in need of convincing or wish to determine your level of fitness, the following tests have been devised as useful indicators and are based on results achieved through testing many thousands of subjects.

Sit ups (described on p. 89)
This is basically an exercise for strengthening the stomach muscles and for the purposes of this test should be performed on the level, with the feet held by a partner or otherwise held in place, e.g. tucked under the bed. Performed at a brisk pace, the following table gives some guide as to your fitness level (figures in brackets are for women): over 70 (35) Excellent; over 50 (25) Very Good; over 40 (20) Good; over 30 (15) Fair; over 20 (10) Average; below 20 (10) Poor.

Berpees or squat thrusts (described on p. 67)
Used as part of the Introduction to Strength and Stamina Routine and also a good test of stamina/muscular endurance. Performed at a brisk pace, the following table is a guide to your fitness level (figures for women in brackets): over 40 (20) Excellent; over 30 (15) Very Good; over 20 (10) Good; over 10 (5) Fair; below 10 (5) Poor.

Step test
Developed in the USA, the (Harvard) Step Test is used as a measure of recovery after exhaustion and involves monitoring the heart's pulse rate at one, two and three minutes after completing a standardised exercise. This consists of stepping up onto a strong gym bench or wooden chair, at a height of 18 inches (.45 metre) (2 in./5 cm lower for women) for a period of 4 minutes (240 seconds). The stepping up and down should be regular and rhythmic.

On completion of the exercise (after 4 minutes) you then take a pulse count for 30 seconds, at intervals of 1, 2 and 3 minutes after finishing the exercise. Make a note of these figures as you will need them to work out the following calculation:

$$\frac{\text{Duration of step test (in seconds)} \times 100}{2 \times \text{sum of three pulse counts}} = \frac{\text{Fitness}}{\text{Rating}}$$

14

Assuming, for example, that your three pulse counts taken after completion of the exercise were 80 (after 1 minute), 65 (after 2 minutes) and 50 (after 3 minutes) the formula would look like this:

$$\frac{240 \text{ (seconds)} \times 100}{2 \times (80 + 65 + 50)} = 61.5$$

According to the Harvard scale this indicates a Fair fitness rating, as the following table shows:

Superior	over 90
Excellent	80–90
Good	70–80
Fair	60–70
Poor	50–60
Very Poor	under 50

Ratings vary according to age, and the above figures are those considered normal for teenagers up to 18, but the test gives a fair indication of your level of fitness, in relation to your heart's ability to return rapidly to normal after raising its pulse rate after exercise. This factor is discussed more fully in a later section when we look at heart and circulation.

Important note
The above pulse rates of 80, 65 and 50 beats per 30 seconds indicate a pulse rate of 160, 130 and 100 beats *per minute* which is fairly high, and the test should not be undertaken by anyone uncertain of their state of health. If you are unable to complete the full four minutes (240 seconds), calculate the time engaged in the exercise and use this figure in working out the formula, for a similarly accurate assessment.

The Need for Exercise

Tests such as those described in the preceding paragraphs have brought to light alarming evidence about the general level of unfitness in Western civilised countries. In Canada, for example, 20% of those tested were considered to have an undesirable fitness level, and a massive 60% achieved only the minimum requirement. Only one fifth of the population were judged to have reached a satisfactory level of fitness and among this group 15% were classed as Good, 4% Very Good and only 1% as Excellent. Tests carried out in the USA during the early 1950s showed an extremely low level of fitness among American children and led to the establishment of the President's Council on Physical Fitness. In later tests British children scored generally better than Americans, but the high incidence of lung cancer and coronary disease (both largely preventable) show that those in adulthood and middle age have largely abandoned the fitness habits practised during youth.

The unfortunate fact is that we are conditioned by the society in which we live to divide our lives into a number of distinct phases after childhood, covering youth and young adulthood, the so-called middle years, and old age. The first period takes us from the age of 20 up to 35 or 40; the second from 40 to 60; and the third from retirement until death. While there is no escape from the inevitability of growing old, these artificial divisions do tend to present a rather depressing picture and help to reinforce the idea that we should automatically 'ease off' after reaching a certain age. There is in fact no justification for this stereotyped attitude.

If we take a naked man aged 25 – at the accepted peak of physical development – and compare him with a naked man of 45, there should be little external physical difference between the two. Provided we take care of our bodies, we are equipped to take part in the same kinds of physical activity at 45 as we are at 25. The fact that we do not or cannot is the result of lack of training and exercise – due of course to factors such as the pressure of work, home, married life and so on. But at least

16

some of our former physical excellence can be recaptured and retained, by a graded programme of exercise.

Even in 'middle age' it is possible to do something about previous years of neglect. At the age of 50, a man can improve his physique by some 75%; at 30 or younger by 100%. And yet most people in their middle years are ten years ahead of their age in terms of bodily decay. Instead, at 40 you can look and feel like 30, and at 30 recover all of the fitness and vigour you experienced at age 20. It *is* possible and this book will show you how.

Most important is to rid the mind of the stereotypes of middle age. Partly perhaps as a result of today's emphasis on youth, reinforced by advertising and the mass media, men in particular are conditioned by attitudes and circumstances to ease off once they get into their thirties, resigning themselves to live out the rest of their lives at something less than half pace.

Meanwhile dissatisfaction with his physical state frequently leads to middle aged depression, sometimes referred to as the male menopause, when men realise they are no longer the lithe, healthy creatures they were in their youth. Sadly the majority of people accept this state of affairs, as though it were inevitable, whereas it is perfectly possible to regain the *fitness image*.

By fitness image we are not talking about super physiques or of people capable of performing great feats of strength or skill, but everyday all-round fitness. Examples abound – among professional sportsmen, actors and others who carry their vigour and youthful looks well into middle age, at a time when most of us are thinking of slowing down and coasting towards old age and retirement.

A system of progressive exercises that makes demands upon the heart, circulation, lungs and the various muscle groups can raise you to a comparable level of fitness that can be *maintained for life*. This means expending a certain amount of time and effort every day, as there are no miracle cures or 'sixty seconds a day is all you need' routines contained in this book. The results however will be positive and beneficial and ultimately lead to a greater enjoyment of life, on a higher plane than you ever dreamed was possible.

Heart & Lungs - the Foundation of Fitness

It is accepted that the basis of any all-round fitness programme must contain elements that by progressive overload-training improve the efficiency of the heart and circulation, and of the lungs and breathing. In order to understand why the efficiency of these organs is vital to our progress it is necessary to study a little of the physiology of the human body. So in this section we look first at the heart and circulation, and later at the lungs and the mechanism of breathing, and study their importance in relation to the development of CR fitness.

Heart

The heart is a powerful muscular organ that beats non-stop throughout our lives, pumping anything between one and five gallons (8–40 pints) of blood per minute (4–22 litres) depending upon the body's require-ment at the time. For its size – no larger than a man's fist and weighing about 14 ounces/.4 kilo – the human heart is an incredibly powerful organ, whose work rate can be further improved by progressive exercise.

At rest the heart of an average adult male beats at between 70 and 80 pulses per minute, pumping about 9 pt/5 l of blood (the body's total capacity) through a series of *arteries* that supply the vital organs and muscles with oxygen. The blood supply returns to the heart through an equally complex network of *veins*.

When we are exercising, the muscles in particular require more oxygen, so that the pulse rate increases – up to 200 or more beats per minute in a very fit person, shifting up to 40 pt/22 l of blood per minute. To cope with the extra demand put upon it, the heart's performance can be improved by progressive exercise, as a result of working it at somewhere near its capacity during training. Because the heart is a muscle it can be strengthened and enlarged, with the result that it beats more powerfully and at a slower rate. As a result the heart of a fit person can have a resting pulse rate of less than 40 beats per minute

18

(common for example among racing cyclists) as opposed to the average rate of 70 beats per minute or more.

The slower basal rate means that the truly fit person can, during exercise, increase his pulse rate fourfold and still be training within safe limits, at about 160–180 beats per minute; whereas an unfit person with a basal rate of 80, by merely doubling this rate is already reaching 160 beats per minute and in an unfit condition this would be an unsafe level at which to train. In any event, it is doubtful if an unfit person could reach this level without difficulty: this would include breathlessness, excessive perspiration and a feeling of giddiness. Longer rest pauses between heart beats mean that the heart works more effectively, reducing the number of beats during the fit person's life *by up to fifty per cent*.

Such a powerful organ as the heart requires its own blood supply, and this reaches the heart by way of two coronary arteries. Exercise improves the performance of the arteries which can become inefficient and when this happens to the coronary artery, parts of the heart may not receive enough oxygen to work efficiently and heart failure may follow. Sharp pains across the chest are among the first signs that all is not well and these warning signs should be heeded and action taken.

Regular exercise will improve the circulation, making the circulatory system into a more efficient transporter of oxygen-rich blood to the organs and muscles (Fig. 1). Where muscles use up more energy than can be supplied by the circulatory system, an *oxygen debt* builds up, leading to aching and cramp as waste products accumulate and are not carried away. This is partly compensated for by the fact that, even when we have finished exercising, the heart continues to beat faster than normal, dealing with the accumulated waste, until recovery is complete. Another effect of improved fitness is this faster rate of recovery, when the pulse returns to normal as was indicated in discussion of the Step Test.

It is not known completely how arteries become clogged with deposits, but causal factors (some of which are discussed elsewhere) include cigarette smoking, a diet that is too rich in animal fats, overweight, high blood pressure and hereditary heart disease. Excess weight and lack of exercise (the two regularly go hand in hand) can also impair circulation through the veins, decreasing the flow of blood back to the heart, a condition known as *venus stasis* (literally 'lazy vein'). Common symptoms are varicose veins in the legs, haemorrhoids and unsightly protruding veins, for example on the forehead.

19

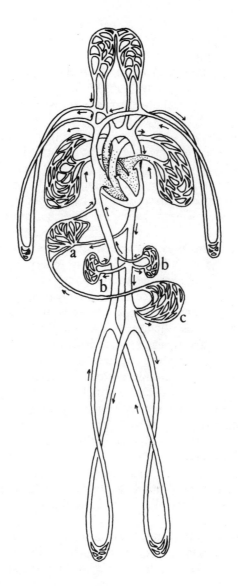

Fig. 1   Circulatory system
Blood is pumped by the heart and carried round the body in a system of arteries
and returned via the veins.
An intricate system of small vessels (capillaries) serves the lungs, to allow for
oxygen/carbon dioxide exchange.
Other organs such as liver (a), kidneys (b) and intestines (c) have their own
supply from branches of the main artery (aorta).

Lungs
We have noted the importance of the heart and circulatory system as a source of oxygen supply vital to the body's functions, and allied to an improvement in the cardio-vascular system must be an increase in the capacity and efficiency of the *lungs*.

The mechanics of breathing are described in Fig. 2. Unfortunately most of us tend to breathe inadequately. This can be the result of poor posture, and because muscles are inactive the capacity of the chest is accordingly reduced. This inevitably leads to breathlessness when we try to exercise.

Air we draw into the lungs is literally the breath of life. The body is composed of millions of living cells which require a constant supply of energy, the source of which is the food we eat. By the process of digestion food is broken down into its constituents, and by a chemical reaction with oxygen these are converted into energy, to keep the body alive and functioning. Waste products are also created, which require efficient removal, and these include water and carbon dioxide.

Along with several other gases and impurities we inhale oxygen when we breathe. The lungs themselves are made up of about 750 million tiny air sacs called *alveoli* which have a combined surface of some 50 square metres (60 sq yds). The air sacs are surrounded by a complex network of blood vessels, and here oxygen enters the bloodstream for transport to all parts of the body, while carbon dioxide is exchanged and enters the lungs, to be exhaled.

Good ventilation of the lungs is therefore necessary, to ensure that an adequate supply of oxygen enters the bloodstream and for getting rid of waste carbon dioxide. The lungs have quite a large air capacity (measured in pints) and total capacity in men is around 10 pints and in women about $7\frac{1}{2}$ pints. We do not always breathe in and out to full capacity and at rest we inhale less than a pint of air with each breath, or some 10 pints per minute.

However, once we start to exercise, the muscles being worked start to burn up more fuel and require more oxygen. As a result we breathe faster, up to 80 breaths a minute, in an attempt to take in more air – inhaling up to 250 pints or more per minute.

Although the action of breathing is largely reflex (it is impossible to suffocate simply by holding your breath) breathing can be controlled. Swimmers learn to do this so that they breathe in time with their strokes, and development of the chest and abdomen through exercise will enhance the capacity of the lungs. Poor chest development leads to shallow breathing, with the result that the lungs are not used to their

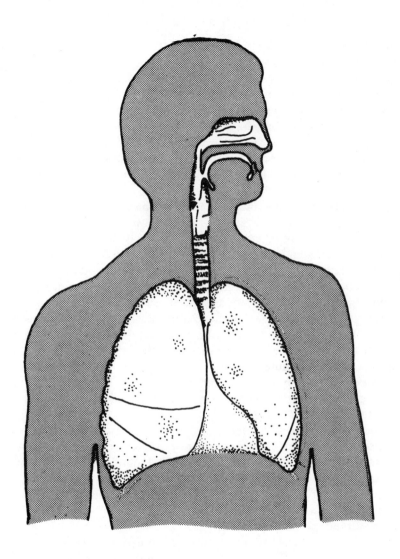

Fig. 2   *The mechanism of breathing*
Air is inhaled through the nose or mouth, and conveyed down the windpipe
(trachea) to the lungs.
There it is trapped inside tiny air sacs (alveoli) which are surrounded by tiny
blood vessels (capillaries). Here oxygen is carried into the blood stream and
carbon dioxide passed into the lungs, to be exhaled.
The diaphragm is a powerful wall of muscle at the foot of the lungs, which separates
the chest cavity from the abdomen. By moving up and down as we breathe,
it controls the capacity of the lungs to inhale and exhale.

full capacity and pockets of stale air remain instead of being exhaled. As a result the succeeding breaths are incomplete and this leads to stagnation and additional strain on the heart and circulation.

A healthy adult can enjoy a chest expansion of several inches (c 16 cm) while practising deep breathing exercises. A number of exercises in this book are designed to improve the size of the chest cavity, allowing the lungs more space in which to work efficiently. A certain amount of breathlessness is experienced during exercise and air may be gulped into the lungs through the mouth. But the fit person will experience a rapid return to normal paced breathing after exertion, leaving the unfit person to collapse with racing heart and panting for breath simply after climbing the stairs or trying to catch a bus.

Regular, progressive exercise will improve the lungs' capacity to draw in more oxygen and the heart's efficiency in delivering it to the body tissues. There, by the process of metabolism, it will be combined with fuel, taken in the form of food we eat, and converted into useful energy. Normal exertion will become comparatively effortless and we will improve our *stamina* – the capacity to keep going during prolonged exercise and shorten the recovery time needed to return to normal. This is the secret of the explosive bursts of energy required by footballers during a hard 90-minute game.

Smoking, which is discussed elsewhere, can seriously damage the delicate air sacs of the lungs and greatly reduce their efficiency. It is sobering to remember that among the over 40s age group, 60 per cent of deaths are due to coronary or respiratory factors.

There are many side effects of fitness, including improved posture and muscle tone, but the key factor is soundness of breathing and circulation – the CR fitness already referred to.

Basic Anatomy

In the chapters dealing with *The need for Exercise* and on the importance of CR fitness as the foundation of any exercise programme, reference has been made to the muscles, as it is by movement of the muscles that useful work is performed and exercise taken. But, before studying the various types of exercises that can form part of a comprehensive fitness programme, it is a good idea to have at least a basic understanding of human anatomy – that is, the study of the body's bone structure (the skeleton), joints and muscles – as this will help you appreciate why certain exercises are undertaken and what is their particular value. This section is therefore a basic introduction to the complex study of human anatomy – starting with the skeleton (Fig. 3).

The human skeleton
The human skeleton forms a framework or scaffold consisting of over 250 bones. To these are attached the muscles which enable the body to move or to hold itself rigid. Where there are two or more bones we find a *joint*. Some joints are immovable but others are designed for a wide range of movement in several planes. Joints are discussed in more detail later. Bones are held together at the joints by *ligaments* and are cushioned against each other by tough gristle or cartilage.

Bones come in a variety of sizes and shapes, from the long bones in the arms and legs, which are light and hollow but extremely strong; to short irregular bones of the type found in the wrists and ankles. Flat circular bones, piled on top of each other and protected by a layer of cartilage, make up the spinal column or back bone. The rib cage, which protects the vital organs of the chest cavity, is made up of round, flattish bones which are themselves attached to the spinal column at the back (the *vertebrae*) and to the breast bone (*sternum*) at the front. The ribs, apart from the two lowest ones, are attached to the breast bone by cartilage, which allows a certain degree of movement when we breathe in and out.

Finally, irregular bones are found, in the skull, where there is no movement other than that of the lower jaw; in the shoulder blades,

24

Fig. 3   *The human skeleton*
(a) *Skull.*
(b) *Collar bone* (clavicle).
(c) *Breast bone* (sternum).
(d) *Shoulder blade* (scapula).
(e) *Bone of upper arm* (humerus).
(f) *Ribs.*
(g) *Back bones* (vertebrae).
(h) *Bones of lower arm* (radius),
and
(i) (ulna).
(j) *Hip bone.*
(k) *Thigh bone* (femur).
(l) *Knee cap* (patella).
(m) *Bones of lower leg* (tibia),
and
(n) (fibula).

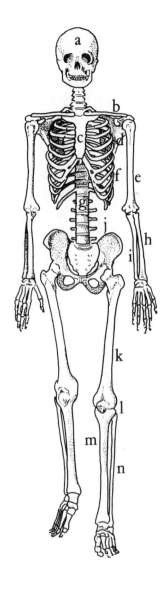

where there are two large triangular shaped bones; and in the pelvic girdle at the base of the trunk, to which the long thigh bone of each leg is connected. A study of the human skeleton will enable you to understand the disposition of the various bones and their functions.

Bones are capable of growth: this accounts for our increase in height and bulk from childhood onwards. Bones are also able to repair themselves if they become broken or cracked (both known as fractures). Another important function of the skeleton concerns the supply of red blood cells (corpuscles) which are formed in the marrow or jelly-like substances that fill the cavities inside certain bones.

Joints

As already noted, where two or more bones meet, they form a joint, and in the context of an exercise programme we are primarily concerned with those joints at which there is movement. The major kinds of movement possible at joints are a swivelling motion, which requires a 'ball and socket' type joint and a hinge movement, such as that possible at the knee and elbow (Fig. 4). Ball and socket joints are found at the shoulders, permitting rotation of the arms through 180° and where the thigh bone joins the pelvic girdle, permitting movement of the legs. Other types of joint are also found, including the gliding or sliding motion of the small bones of the wrist and ankle, and the pivoting motion between the skull and the top of the spinal column that allows us to move the head in several directions.

Bones are held together at joints by cartilage and, to facilitate movement, are encased in a (synovial) membrane that secretes a fluid that acts as a lubricant between the bony surfaces. At the powerful knee joint, the area is protected by the 'knee cap' and well cushioned by cartilage.

Joints are designed only for their own particular type of movement and where injuries occur at joints they are known as dislocations; the bones are pulled apart unnaturally and there is usually damage to the ligaments and surrounding muscle tissues.

Muscles

Equipped with just the bony structure of the skeleton and the freedom of movement allowed by certain joints we are still unable to move our bodies without the aid of muscles. And it is towards the development of our muscles, so that they are capable of doing more work, that much of our fitness programme is directed.

There are over 650 muscles in the body and of these the skeletal muscles enable the limbs and other parts of the body to move by a system of expansion and contraction. Other muscles surround and protect the

26

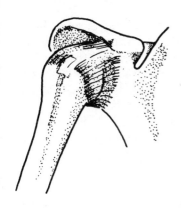

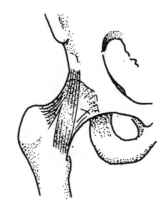

(a) *Ball and socket joint at shoulder.*   (b) *Ball and socket joint at hip.*

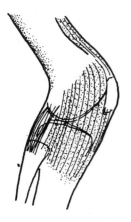

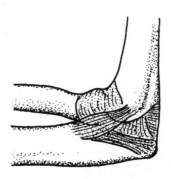

(c) *Hinge joint at knee.*   (d) *Hinge joint at elbow.*

Fig. 4   *Common types of joints*

internal organs and in the case of the heart do useful work themselves. Muscles are made of tough stringy tissues that require a copious blood supply and they are capable of growth and development. They are attached to the bones by means of *tendons* which are tough strands similar to the *ligaments* that keep bones together at the joints.

Muscles are arranged in groups and invariably work in pairs. When one muscle contracts (it is then known as the 'prime mover') it requires the assistance of a second muscle (called the 'antagonist') to allow it to then relax. To do this, the antagonist (now the prime mover) contracts while the first muscle (now the antagonist) relaxes, and so on. The way muscles work is shown in the accompanying illustration.

In order to understand the principle of exercise, including working with weights, you should be familiar with the major muscle groups of the Arms and Shoulders, Trunk and Legs.

Arms and shoulders
Powerful muscles are at work here enabling us to lift and carry. The *deltoids* allow movement of the arm, while the upper arm itself consists of two major muscles – the *biceps* to the front and the *triceps* to the rear (Fig. 5).

Trunk
High across lie the *pectoral* muscles and below these the *abdominals* cushioning the vital organs of the stomach and digestive tract. These together with the *intercostal* muscles can be developed to give the impressive 'washboard' type of abdomen.

Legs
The front of the thigh consists of a number of extremely powerful muscles responsible for moving the legs in running, kicking, weight training, etc. They include the *quadriceps* group; and at the rear, the *hamstring* group. High up, forming the seat, are the *gluteals*. Two sections of muscle make up the calves – the two heads of the *gastrocnemius* muscles (popularly known as the 'gastros') and, to the front, the *tibialis anterior* helps manipulate the foot.

These muscles and others are illustrated in Fig. 6.

Muscles can be exercised progressively, enabling them to do more work – lifting, running, etc. – without suffering undue strain. By increasing their size, their energy production capacity is improved, so that more work can be handled without the build-up of an oxygen debt causing aches and discomfort. It is essential that any increase in work load is gradual and progressive, otherwise damage to muscle tissue can occur or, at best, you will suffer from stiffness and strains. It is also important to warm-up before engaging in physical activity.

Any development of the skeletal muscles will quickly improve the outline shape of the body, by improving muscle line and definition and

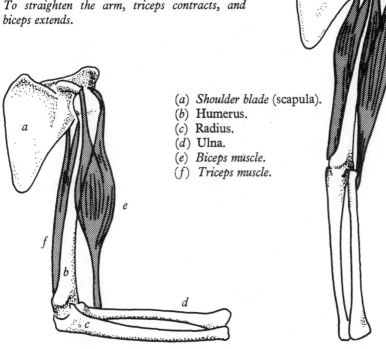

Fig. 5   The mechanics of movement
Muscles of the upper arm (shaded) show how movement is accomplished as muscles work in pairs. As the arm is bent (e.g. to perform a curl), biceps muscle contracts and triceps is extended. To straighten the arm, triceps contracts, and biceps extends.

(a) *Shoulder blade* (scapula).
(b) Humerus.
(c) Radius.
(d) Ulna.
(e) *Biceps muscle.*
(f) *Triceps muscle.*

generally enhancing the physique. There will also be a notable improvement in posture. Because the shoulders are pulled back and the stomach muscles strengthened, unsightly abdominal sag is eliminated at the same time as inches are trimmed off the waist.

However, it should be noted that no amount of exercise will alter your basic *body type*. Although every human being is different, certain characteristics enable physiques to be classified into three major groups: endomorph, mesomorph and ectomorph. The endomorph is characterised by roundness and relatively short stature and although well muscled the outline tends to be obscured by layers of flesh that are not so apparent on the mesomorph. The mesomorph, popularly regarded as the ideal for the all-round sportsman, has typically broad shoulders and narrow waist, the type of physique on which muscular development

29

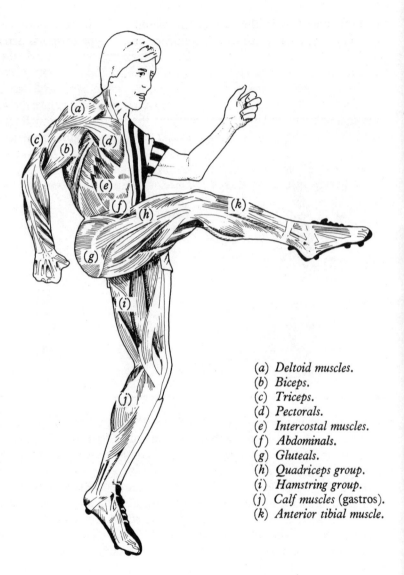

(a) *Deltoid muscles.*
(b) *Biceps.*
(c) *Triceps.*
(d) *Pectorals.*
(e) *Intercostal muscles.*
(f) *Abdominals.*
(g) *Gluteals.*
(h) *Quadriceps group.*
(i) *Hamstring group.*
(j) *Calf muscles* (gastros).
(k) *Anterior tibial muscle.*

Fig. 6 *Major muscle groups*

quickly produces dramatic improvements in shape and definition. The ectomorph in contrast is typically skinny, with shoulders and hips the same width. Muscle bulk can be added but progress will not be so rapid or pronounced as in the case of the mesomorph. Some experts claim that body type has considerable influence on the type of sports activity undertaken, as most top class athletes (all sports) tend towards meso-ectomorphy, although shot putters and others come from the ranks of the endomorphs. It is claimed that the pure ectomorph tends towards track events, particularly marathon and cross-country running where his characteristic independence confirms the image of the loneliness of the long distance runner. This contrasts dramatically with the generally open and gregarious nature of the typical endomorph and mesomorph, which makes them ideal participants in team sports of all kinds.

Body type cannot be altered but all-round fitness can be achieved by everyone.

Food

We have already noted that in order to perform work the muscles require a source of energy, this is supplied in the form of the food we eat. The energy from food is released by means of a chemical process, rather like burning, during which oxygen is consumed and carbon dioxide and other waste products produced. Even at rest the body requires a certain level of energy in order to continue functioning, and the higher the workload, through exercise for example, the greater will be its energy/fuel requirement. This is normally supplied by consuming a balanced diet – one that not only supplies the necessary quantity and bulk, but also contains the numerous minerals and other elements vital for our survival.

Fuel for the body
The *quantity* of food we consume should be closely related to our need and this will vary according to our lifestyle. A person leading a sedentary life, working in an office for example, will have a smaller requirement than a heavy manual worker who uses more physical energy during the course of a day. The secret of dietary balance is to match food input to energy output as closely as possible, in order to avoid the excess weight gain which results from eating more food than the body can use.

The body's energy requirement is measured in Calories. Even at rest, it requires a certain amount of energy (known as basal metabolism) simply to maintain the heart and circulation, and permit breathing and functioning of other vital organs in order to keep the body alive. At rest an average man requires about 1600 Calories daily in order to stay alive.

Once we start to move and work or take exercise, the body's Calorie requirement increases and we need to eat more than the basic 1600 Calories per day. Human beings are not identical and some people appear to use up energy faster than others, but *average* daily requirements can be assessed. The energy value of food is also expressed in

Calories and a glance at the tables on page 112 will quickly give you an idea of the calorific value of a number of popular foods.

Once we have established the calorific value of the food we eat, we can match it to our energy requirements. We have noted already that basal metabolism requires some 1600 Calories daily. To get us through a normal day the average man needs to take in a further 1000 Calories (total 2600), slightly less for a woman; teenagers, who are still growing and more active physically, will require rather more, say a further 500 Calories; while elderly or retired people, unless they are very active, probably need around 2300 daily Calories or less.

Once we start to engage in serious physical activity, either hard manual work or a programme of exercise, the body's Calorie requirements rise dramatically – to 3500 Calories or more per day. Energy expenditure is also measured in Calories and as a guide, jogging for an hour will consume some 500 Calories and a 90-minute game of football will consume around 1000 or more. Even a brisk walk will use up some 300 Calories per hour.

By matching our food intake to the amount of energy we expend we can achieve a fairly precise balance between Calories consumed and Calories expended. Failure to strike the correct balance will result in accumulation of surplus fat and serious problems of overweight or, in the case of under-eating, it will lead to loss of weight and a general feeling of lethargy.

To lose excess weight, therefore, it should be clear that the simple formula is to eat less and exercise more with the result that the body uses more Calories than it consumes and starts to use up some of the reserves it has stored in the form of excess fat. Once we reach the required level (by consulting the ideal Height/Weight chart on page 117) we can revert to a normal diet.

A sensible slimming diet will attempt to reduce the number of Calories consumed, while continuing to provide nutrition and variety. The ideal slimming diet will be composed of fewer fats and carbohydrates ('filler' foods) but will contain sufficient protein, minerals and vitamins for tissue growth and repair.

There is really no mystery about slimming diets and although numerous artificial aids are available on the market, the phrase 'Calorie controlled diet' means no more than it says: to lose weight you must control the number of Calories you consume.

Vitamins, proteins, minerals and carbohydrates
We are concerned not only with consuming the right quantity of food

(measured in Calories) but also with eating a balanced diet that contains the number of essential elements needed to maintain the body processes and encourage growth and repair of body tissue. Foods are classified according to their main constituents – as follows:

Carbohydrates and fats
The rich energy producing Calorie-loaded foods, including most starches, sugars etc.

Proteins
Long–term energy producers, providing the essential amino acids required to keep the body alive. Found in meat, eggs, fish, cheese, peanuts etc.

Vitamins
Found in traces in many foods and classified under 17 headings – Vitamins A, B1 to B12, C, D, E and K.

Vitamin A is found in carrots, egg yolk, liver, butter and most green vegetables and is important for good sight. Vitamins B1–B12 are found in a variety of foods, including whole-meal flour, bacon, egg yolk (B1), cheese, liver, ham, tomatoes (B2) and so on. Vitamin C helps the body to fight infection and promotes healing and growth and is found mainly in fresh fruit, and in specially manufactured Vitamin C substances – tablets, powder etc.

Various minerals, including iron, calcium, phosphates, sodium and potassium are also needed in minute daily quantities and are contained in some foods (meat, some fresh vegetables, milk etc).

Without becoming a slave to any particular diet, care should be taken that sufficient quantities of the correct foods are eaten daily. Broadly speaking, this means eating one or more of the items from each of the following groups every day: this will provide the correct balance of nutrients in the form of vitamins, proteins and minerals for normal requirements:

Group A   Cheese and milk
Group B   Meat, fish, eggs
Group C   Fresh fruit and vegetables
Group D   Butter or margarine

To these must be added the energy giving foods, in the form of carbo-hydrates (bread, potatoes, pastry, cakes, sugar etc.).

Fatigue, Rest, Sleep and Relaxation

The really fit person is rarely troubled with insomnia, and once you have started on your exercise programme you will find yourself falling asleep more naturally and awaking refreshed.

The amount of sleep we require varies from one person to another and according to age. Newly born babies sleep most of the time and young children need up to twelve hours. Teenagers who are developing rapidly require 8 to 10 hours sleep, while adults usually need 7 to 8 hours – occasionally less.

There is no scientific evidence to support the theory that sleep before midnight is more beneficial (i.e. 'an hour before midnight is worth two after' is simply not true) and provided we get enough sleep for our personal requirements we should not be troubled by insomnia or tiredness. There are varying depths of sleep, and the deepest period occurs within 30 to 60 minutes of our falling asleep, becoming lighter by degrees until we wake up seven or eight hours later. The pattern is illustrated in Fig. 7.

Dreams occur during the periods of lighter sleep. Everyone dreams but not all of us can remember them. During the periods of deepest sleep, which last for two to three hours, muscles are relaxed and pulse rate and body temperature are lowered.

Apart from resting during sleep, it is sometimes beneficial to relax during the day, even 'catnapping', provided this is not done to excess i.e. to the detriment of regular sleep at night. One of the many side benefits of exercise is the ability to relax easily and naturally, without resort to mysticism or the more esoteric Oriental philosophies. Mental and physical stress resulting from work, an unsatisfactory home situation, a bereavement etc. can all contribute to tension, which can be manifested in a number of ways: insomnia, stomach complaints, lack of appetite, a vague feeling of being run down or unable to cope. People who are tired and tense quickly become impatient, irritable and subject to anxiety and depression, all of which can rapidly affect their work and home life.

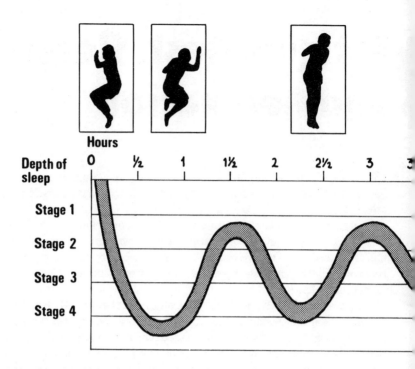

Fig. 7　*The stages of sleep*
We gradually fall asleep within half an hour and then enjoy our deepest sleep
(Stage 4). As the night progresses sleep becomes lighter until awaking. Dreams
occur during Stage 2 sleep mainly, and often last for as long as 45 minutes.

While exercise will not make your problems go away, the achievement
of physical goals and the participation in exercise and sport bring satis-
faction and relief from tension. At the same time, increased strength and
stamina make you better able to cope with the stresses and strains of
daily life.

Sound sleep requires both physical and mental fatigue. Too many
people go to bed feeling mentally exhausted, but fail to sleep well
because they are not physically tired.

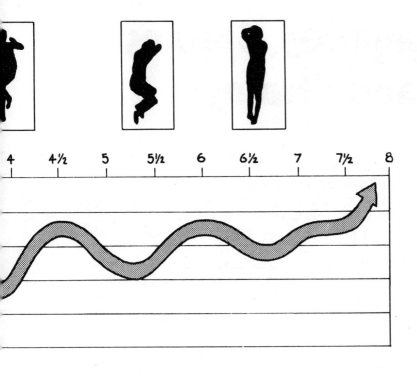

4 4½ 5 5½ 6 6½ 7 7½ 8

Injuries, Sprains and Strains

Anyone taking up exercise after a long lay-off can expect to experience some aches and pains, when for the first time strain is put on muscles, ligaments and joints that have not been exercised for years. You must expect them to require a little time to adjust to the new demands placed upon them.

Without becoming a hypochondriac, *pain should never be ignored*. Pain should not be masked by using pain killing (analgesic) drugs or sprays for local application. The source of the pain should be located and appropriate action taken. Temporary relief of the muscular pain associated with exercise can sometimes be achieved by the use of cold compresses or the application of heat as appropriate. All athletic activity produces some stiffness and soreness and much of this can be 'worked off' by more exercise. However, serious or protracted pain should not be ignored and medical advice should be sought at the earliest opportunity.

Running and jogging can produce soreness in the calves and thigh muscles, while training with weights can also strain arm, shoulder, chest, back and stomach muscles. These slight aches will normally wear off during your rest day and should not cause problems provided you remember to warm up correctly before each exercise session and finish with a relaxing bath or hot shower.

Strains and sprains should be clearly distinguished. *Strains* result from the over-stretching or tearing of muscle fibre and usually produce pain and swelling in the affected area, with occasional bruising. Rest and the application of cold compresses to reduce the swelling are the normal treatment. *Sprain* describes an injury to the area of *joints*, usually the result of severe wrenching and consequent damage to tendons and possibly to surrounding tissues and blood vessels. Where the bones are displaced *dislocation* has occurred, and movement of the joint may be impossible or extremely painful. Medical advice should be sought at once.

Pulled muscles are the result of damage or injury where the muscle and tendon join, injuries to the hamstrings being comparatively common in sport. Stretching and warm-up routines *before* exercising will help to prevent this condition, which can result in prolonged treatment and a lay-off of two months or more.

Progressive exercise strengthens muscles and causes them to grow in size, with the result that they can be worked harder. Stiffness results when waste products are not shifted fast enough, but exercise will improve muscle tone and enhance the circulatory system with the result that prolonged exercise will become gradually easier.

A common complaint among joggers and runners is buck shin or shin splints. The symptoms are pain and stiffness around the shin bone, due to slight tearing of the connective tissue. Frequently, the cause is running on hard pavements, as opposed to soft ground. This can also cause strain to the Achilles tendon at the rear of the ankle. Correct warm-up, stretching exercises and the use of thick–soled shoes can help avoid the condition.

Because the knee joint has to do a large amount of work it is particularly susceptible to injury and any sudden or sharp twisting can dislodge the cartilages that cushion the bones of the knee joint. The usual result is total collapse of the knee, as it buckles under the weight of the sportsman. Strengthening the muscles of the inner and outer aspects of the thigh will do much to avoid knee injuries: these must include squats (for the outer thigh) and leg extensions (for the inner) to provide a correct balance of strength at this joint. Cycling either on a stationary exerciser or on a bicycle is an excellent way of strengthening these muscles without unduly straining the knee joint.

Tennis elbow is the name given to a variety of pains and swelling in the forearm that can result from too vigorous exercise, either through playing sports or from such activities as sawing wood. The normal cure involves resting the affected part, and medical advice must be sought if the pain is severe or prolonged.

Groin strain is harder to define. Pain is usually felt down the inside of the thigh and occasionally as an ache in the testicles and groin region overall. Once again, lay-off, rest and analgesics are the usual forms of treatment, and medical advice should be sought.

Fractures (breaking or partial damage to a bone) should not normally occur in non-contact sports. The best preventive measure for all types of injuries is correct warm-up and correct technique, particularly when handling weights and other apparatus.

Smoking and Alcohol

An analysis of the ten leading causes of death in western countries shows that the most common killers are: heart disease, cancer, accidents, strokes, influenza, bronchitis, pneumonia, diabetes, cirrhosis, injuries or malformation at birth, and suicide. What is significant about this list is that many of the causes are largely *preventable* and in many cases are aggravated by lack of exercise, and over-indulgence in food, alcohol and tobacco.

Where our health is concerned, absolutely nothing can be said in favour of smoking. A glance at statistics will quickly explain why. Cigarette smokers are twice as likely to die during middle age as non-smokers; every year in the U.K. over twenty thousand deaths in men aged between 35 and 65 are caused by smoking; and the chances are that *two out of five* heavy smokers will die before the age of 65.

Of the main components in a cigarette, many are toxic. These include hydrogen cyanide, ammonia, carbon monoxide, nicotine, butane, phenol and tar, and in the inexperienced smoker these substances can produce feelings of dizziness, nausea, vomiting, heightened pulse rate and cold sweat. Although these symptoms disappear with experience, the damage done increases, as tiny particles of nicotine and other substances used in the manufacture of cigarettes are inhaled and cling to the delicate alveoli of the lungs and eventually enter the bloodstream.

As a result, the number of diseases known to be closely linked to smoking includes heart and arterial conditions, chronic bronchitis, gastric and duodenal ulcers, tuberculosis of the lungs, diseases of the mouth and gums and of course lung cancer.

The sportsman who smokes puts himself at a serious disadvantage, impairing his bodily efficiency while asking his body to perform at its maximum. The likelihood is that a serious programme of exercise will encourage you to give up smoking altogether.

Addiction to alcohol is only slightly less pernicious than addiction to nicotine. All alcohol is poisonous to some degree and, because it has a

Calorie content, it can supply up to one–fifth of the body's energy requirements without providing essential nutrients. As a result, carbohydrates and fats taken in normal food tend to be deposited in the tissues as surplus fat. Alcohol acts as a *depressant* rather than as a stimulant as it impairs the efficiency of the central nervous system through its anaesthetic action.

Although moderate amounts of alcohol have a useful side effect in stimulating the secretions of the stomach and therefore aiding digestion, excess intake of alcohol can seriously irritate the mucous membrane lining of the stomach and lead to chronic indigestion, as well as cirrhosis of the liver.

Exercise Routines

The exercises are designed to provide the maximum amount of variety to achieve all-round fitness and allow the reader to work with weights, to train indoors or out, to work alone or with a partner. They are classified into Warm-up (these routines should always be performed before any session by all grades) and exercises for the four main areas of the body – Arms/Shoulders, Chest, Stomach/Back and Legs.

Unfit*
Perform the warm-up routines only for a period of two weeks, with three exercise sessions each week (more frequently if desired and no strain is felt). This should be followed by a further period, say two weeks, of the Introduction to Strength and Stamina routines (one star level). After 4 weeks of this preparation, you should attempt a *selection* of exercises from each major group. If you intend to use weights, try a few sessions performing the movement only (without weights) and then proceed to a light weight that you can comfortably handle. The repetitions should be as stated for Unfit and it is likely that you will remain at this level for 6 to 8 weeks before moving on to the Medium Fit grade.

Medium Fit**
Perform the warm-up routines before every session. Strength and Stamina exercises may be used at any time. Selected exercises are then performed from each of the major groups, with the correct number of repetitions followed. Only when you are handling suggested poundages and repetitions comfortably and for a period of not less than 6 weeks should you take the step up to Superfit. (If after a trial this grade appears too advanced, revert to Medium for a few weeks and try again.)

Superfit***
Perform the warm-up routines before every session. Strength and Stamina exercises may be performed at any time. Selected exercises are

then taken from the major groups, observing recommended poundages and numbers of repetitions. Poundages are progressively increased.

It is not intended that all the exercises illustrated should be attempted in one session. They are designed to provide all-round movement, utilising the major muscle groups, and to provide variation according to circumstances. Many of the movements are duplicated, using a free-standing action, weights, your own or partner's body-weight and so on. You should select the ones suited to your circumstances.

It is important to select exercises from each group, with a minimum of *five* being performed from each of the four major groups, making a session of some 20 exercises, plus the initial warm-up routines. Avoid the temptation to concentrate on certain body areas, for example, thighs, while neglecting the arms. Go for overall development.

The routines can be combined with running, football or other sports activity and it is suggested that three sessions a week (with other activities in between) will produce the best results.

Your Exercise Schedule

When and how often should you exercise?

Obviously there are certain times when you should *not* exercise and these include too soon after eating. It is advisable to leave three to four hours clear between finishing a meal and undertaking any serious training such as jogging or weights. It is also suggested that you wait for an hour or two after completing training before eating a meal, allowing time for the system to 'wind down' to normal.

As to the best time of day to train, this depends to some extent upon opportunity and finding the optimum time that suits your system, a time at which you feel at your best. This can be early morning, particularly if you train out of doors, when the air is sweeter and if you are in town you avoid at least the worst of the traffic pollution. Alternatively some people may prefer to train during the lunchtime period (though this will mean foregoing lunch itself), others during the late afternoon or early evening.

The frequency of exercise will depend on your initial state of fitness and how far you are progressing in your own schedule. 'Little and often' is better than exercise taken in great bursts, with prolonged rest periods in between. You can certainly exercise daily, with some variation in the actual routine, for example, jogging one day, using weights the next. Serious weight training sessions are usually three times a week, with a rest day in between to allow for local recovery of the muscles worked. Once you make progress into your schedule it is hard to allow yourself a day off and most people end up training daily.

Obviously you should not rush into any exercise programme but work into it gently. You should not exercise if you are feeling unwell and correct warming up procedure should help you to avoid sprains and strains.

Planning an Exercise Schedule

Whenever you watch a football game you will notice that the players trot out onto the pitch some five minutes before the game is due to begin. As well as kicking a ball round and getting the feel of the ground, they perform a number of stretching movements with the trunk and legs; touching the toes, high kicks, sideways splits and so on. These are all designed to warm up the body for exertion and improve mobility and, even for the highly trained player, they are an essential preliminary to any form of serious exercise.

For the unfit person, it would clearly be foolish suddenly to subject an unaccustomed body to a crash programme of hard physical work, without some kind of prior preparation. Every doctor will tell you about his annual crop of early spring casualties, of strained backs and aching limbs at the start of the gardening season or when hundreds of sedentary individuals shake off their winter lethargy and try their first game of tennis.

It follows, therefore, that a considerable section of this book is devoted to warm-up exercise routines. For the totally unfit they are an essential preparation for more serious training. And even when we have got the body into reasonable shape, at least some of these exercises should be performed as a preliminary warm-up, to boost the circulation, loosen up joints and help prevent muscular aches and strains. This applies to football or tennis matches, jogging sessions, skiing, gymnastics – any serious exercise session. *Your warm-up routines should never be omitted.*

With the body reasonably tuned-up it is now ready for some real physical work. Again without using any special kinds of apparatus, a whole range of *free-standing* exercises can be performed to improve strength and stamina. They include such movements as the press-up, squats, star jumps, sit-ups, berpees and many others which are described fully on the appropriate pages.

By working with a partner or in a small group, other exercises can be introduced that make use of the partner's body weight, such as a pick-a-back, alternate partner raising and so on. And by the addition of even very basic equipment the whole range of movements can be enlarged, by introducing barbells, dumbells, springs and some form of exercise bench. By using this sort of equipment the body starts to pit its strength against resistance.

There are numerous exercises that can be performed with weights and it is advisable to be clear from the outset about the difference between 'weight training' and 'body building'. There is also the science of 'weight lifting', but this is in reality a separate sport, carried out to Olympic standards. Body building is another specialised activity, in which participants aim to increase muscle size and definition as an end in itself, using very high poundages and generally slow and infrequent repetitions.

If you are aiming at *all-round fitness* – and that is the purpose of this book – then weight *training* can be used. This consists of using weight lifting apparatus – basically the barbell and dumbells – with the emphasis on moderate weight that you can comfortably shift at a fairly fast pace. The poundage is gradually increased to provide the muscles being exercised with more and more work to do. The gradual increases in weight are achieved by adding extra metal plates or discs to the dumbell or barbell.

Other gymnasium apparatus includes the exercise bench, either flat or sloping, that is used in many pressing and lifting motions, as well as sit-ups (on an incline). There are also special pieces of apparatus designed to exercise the calf muscles, shoulder muscles, abdominals etc., but the principle behind all these pieces of equipment is the same; to enable the user to exercise certain muscles in the optimum position and avoid strain. For example a heavier weight bench press can be performed if the weight (barbell) is lowered onto the exerciser by an assistant or first placed onto a special stand behind the bench while the exerciser gets into position.

It is possible to buy a set of weights and exercise at home. Starting poundages will vary according to your state of fitness and you should not try to shift more weight than you can comfortably handle. If muscles seriously ache after a trial session you have probably been trying to do too much. A fairly large floor area is required, particularly if you intend to add benches etc. Alternatively you can join a weight training club or gym, where you could attend two or three times a week, and perform exercises with apparatus under supervision.

In this book the minimum of specialised equipment is used to illustrate the various exercises and use is frequently made of everyday objects

46

(such as a park bench) that can be adapted to assist in performing certain routines.

Another useful piece of apparatus that you can either use at home or take with you when travelling is the chest expander. This is a device made of metal springs or tough rubber strands, that are attached to handles; more springs/strands can be added to vary the amount of effort needed to stretch them. Many of the movements achieved by lifting weights can be simulated using the springs and where appropriate these are illustrated in the exercise routines.

A doorway bar can complete your home gym equipment. This is designed to fit into a doorway opening and can be used for all kinds of pull-up and hanging exercises, which strengthen muscles and ease the load on the spine; hanging for a few minutes after exercising helps to separate the vertebrae of the spinal column by traction.

It is not essential then that a progressive exercise schedule need involve the purchase of any specialised equipment, and the use of weights and other apparatus by the reader can be regarded purely as an optional extra, to which he might progress at a later stage or use to introduce variety into his routines. There are no new or undiscovered forms of exercise shown in this book and many of the basic routines such as the press-up or the sit-up will doubtless be familiar. They are however the foundation of any serious exercise schedule that aims to make demands on the lungs and circulation and improve the tone and definition of the surface muscles. They can be performed on your own, in the privacy of your home, at any time to suit your convenience. It is not necessary to invest in any specialised apparatus.

What to Wear for Exercise

Some sports obviously have their own special clothing – football shorts and jerseys, a tennis outfit, cricket pads and gloves, and so on. But for most other exercise activities such as weight training or jogging, you require only simple clothing that will keep you reasonably warm and allow complete freedom of movement.

For indoor work (and outdoors in warm weather) your outfit can consist of the following: cotton vest or T-shirt; cotton or wool socks and light pumps or plimsols. Men should support their genitals either with brief underpants or a jock strap. Your outfit should be easily washable.

For outdoor work you can add a warmer top like an old jersey or track suit jacket, and in cold weather track suit trousers or tights should be worn, and for really cold days these can be complemented by warm long underpants, woollen gloves or mits and a woollen hat.

When the body becomes cold, blood tends to drain from the extremities – hands, feet, surface flesh – to concentrate additional supplies to the vital organs. It is essential to warm-up (in both senses) before exercising and retain this warmth, without undue perspiring. The warm clothing will prevent heat loss, particularly through the scalp (some 60 per cent) when a woollen hat is worn.

If you get too warm while exercising, some clothing may be discarded as the body will otherwise have to work extra hard, through sweating, to regulate your temperature to a lower, more acceptable level. Afterwards warm clothing should be replaced until you take a bath or shower on completion of the session.

Particular care should be taken that the correct type of shoes are worn for road work – jogging, distance running, sprints. Because of the fashion in shoes with fairly high heels among young people, the Achilles tendon can become shortened and a sudden switch to flat-soled exercise shoes will produce unaccustomed stretching that may cause eventual injury. The avoidance of excessively high heels is therefore to be recommended, coupled with adequate warm-up and stretching routines before starting to exercise. A sponge rubber pad inserted under the heels inside running shoes will take some of the harshness out of prolonged road work and help to cushion the impact of the heel on the hard ground.

Although any old clothes can be worn for exercising, smart new kit, of the correct type and fit is preferable. Your whole appearance will be more professional. It goes without saying of course that all training kit should be frequently washed and kept in good repair.

The Body's Cooling Mechanism

Once our muscles start to work during exercise, energy is burnt up and heat generated – and it is at this point that the body's heat regulating mechanisms move into action. Some of the phenomena connected with temperature control are already familiar to us, and these include sweating, dilation of the blood vessels and a glow or flush over the surface of the skin. Why do these manifestations occur?

Sweating or perspiration is an excretion through the pores of the skin, 98% liquid but containing traces of salts. In normal activity we lose up to 1 pint (570 ml) of sweat daily but in hot climates or during excessive physical activity this figure can rise dramatically, to as much as 15 pt/8.5 l daily sweat loss. The action of sweating is an important cooling mechanism, when sweat evaporates from the skin on exposure to the air. During profuse sweating through exertion or high outside temperature, sweat pours from the skin in droplets and no cooling effect is produced.

We do not perspire equally in all regions of the body as sweat glands tend to be concentrated in certain areas, such as the palms of the hands and soles of the feet.

Another heat regulating mechanism is the increase in size of the blood vessels that occurs during exertion. This exposes more surface blood vessels to the external air and in turn aids a reduction in body heat. Flushing is a similar reaction of the nervous system, acting on minute capillary vessels.

Fresh perspiration in normal health is without smell and body odour only occurs when stale perspiration remains on the skin and reacts with the bacteria present on the skin surface. So a shower taken straight after exercise and frequent changes of clothing should avoid the problem.

What Should You Weigh?

All foods have a Calorie value and the more energy the body uses up the greater will be its Calorie requirement. If we take on board more Calories than we need the result is an accumulation of fatty tissue composed of the excess food consumed that has not been used up by the proper expenditure of energy.

To lose weight, therefore, all that is needed is to consume fewer Calories than we burn up, with the result that with exercise we use up our reserves of fat and excess weight is shed from the body. *There are no easy routes to weight reduction* and although some so-called crash diets may produce dramatic results during the first few days, they are not recommended for general or continuous use and should not be undertaken without medical supervision.

A sensible slimming diet will simply cut down the number of Calories (to between 1200 and 1500 daily), while continuing to provide a balance of nutrition and variety. The slimming diet will have to contain sufficient protein to build and repair body tissues and provide some energy, and fewer fats and carbohydrates which are 'filler' foods and loaded with Calories. You will also need a regular intake of essential vitamins, minerals and salts and these are obtained in any normal diet, particularly where the accent is on raw/fresh fruit and vegetables.

Hunger pangs can be allayed by taking warm drinks or clear soup and you can eat plenty of salads for bulk. Certain drugs used to be prescribed as appetite depressants but many of them are now considered to be addictive. Artificial sweeteners can however be used in place of sugar.

Without becoming an obsessive Calorie counter there are certain foods that the slimmer will obviously try to avoid. You know almost instinctively what these are: they include pastries, puddings, pies, bread, potatoes, fats, chocolates, ice cream and a whole variety of manufactured foods (pizza, pasta etc.) with a high Calorie content. In place of these you can revert to the basics such as lean meat and poultry, fish, eggs, plain cheeses, milk, yoghurt, fresh fruit and vegetables and salads.

51

Some foods should be avoided almost always, because of their high Calorie content and these include pastry (1200 Calories per 8 ounces) and double cream (1300 per $\frac{1}{2}$-pint carton). Milk is quite high in Calories (370 per pint) and the allowance taken in tea, coffee etc. should be included in your daily reckoning.

It can be noted in passing that liquids should be taken normally during a slimming diet. Methods of inducing excessive perspiration such as sauna or Turkish baths will produce immediate weight loss, but as the resultant thirst is satisfied with something to drink the pounds return.

Fitness and Sex

Among the popular myths associated with sex is the belief that sexual activity is somehow weakening, and conversely that certain exercises or foods or drugs will enhance sexual performance.

A number of authorities have conducted surveys among top-class athletes and the conclusions arrived at are that normal sexual activity can be conducted right through any sort of training programme, up to and including the night before the big event, provided that one is getting the usual quota of restful sleep.

The only factors that will help to make you fit sexually are the same ones that apply to fitness generally; exercise, fresh air, correct diet, sleep – and a balanced attitude to the whole subject.

Running

Running is an important part of many fitness training programmes. Many team games are based around frequent stops and starts – explosive bursts followed by a few seconds recovery. To train for this sort of activity calls for the introduction of short sprints, backwards sprinting, sideways running and other movements designed to improve stamina and reduce recovery time.

Running exercises large groups of muscles, including the calves, thighs and abdomen. In addition, increased demand is put on the heart and lungs, and included in the side benefits is the certainty that you will lose excess fat, particularly from around the waist. The demand for oxygen that this activity will generate ensures that lungs are used to their full capacity and chest development improved.

Running over fairly long distances – 1 to 10 miles/1.6 – 17 km – at a slow pace (also known as jogging) can be used as a fitness programme in itself, provided that it is progressive. You need either to increase the distance covered or the speed at which you run – or both. It is possible to jog at any age and as often as you wish; many advocates jog daily.

All running demands an efficient style that will not cause unnecessary strain. The most popular is the heel-to-toe method; you land first on the heel and then rock forward onto the ball of the foot. You then spring forward using the toes to give leverage, as you go into your next pace (Fig. 8).

If you find that you are running incorrectly – and excessive soreness will be among the telltale signs – your style can be improved as you learn to 'give' more at the knees, enabling you to land with a full foot on the ground. The temptation to land on the toes results from wearing shoes with built-up heels and a period of adjustment to flat soles is required, as more strain is put on the Achilles tendon.

Distance running need not be competitive and a fast pace is not necessary; aim to cover one mile/1.6 km in anything from 6 to 15 minutes. You can gradually increase the distance covered at each outing, starting with half a mile/.4 km or less, rising to 5 miles/8 km or more.

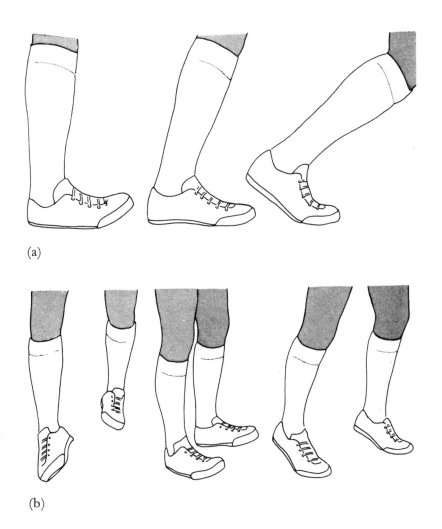

Fig. 8   Running styles
(a) Heel-to-toe method of running.
(b) Additional exercises include walking on the side of the foot, heels and toes.

To gain additional leg power and improve stamina you should not confine your running to distance outings at a measured rhythmic pace. Some variety should be introduced, including sprints, hill running, speed bursts, interval running etc., as described in the following exercises.

Conditioning programme
A 2 to 3 mile/3 – 5 km slow run (jog), followed by 10 fast paced interval runs; run the length of a soccer pitch at a fast pace, then walk back and repeat 10 times.

Sprint bursts
Using a soccer pitch perimeter or similar, cover the total distance in a mixture of fast sprints (about 30 yds/27 m each) interspersed with jogs for recovery.

Combination run
Use a measured distance of 3 to 4 miles/5 – 6.5 km. This is covered by a 1 mile jog/1.6 km; the second mile/1.6 km – sprint bursts (max 50 yds/45 m) (5 or 6) with a jog for recovery in between each one; $\frac{1}{2}$ mile/.8 km recovery jog; $\frac{1}{4}$ mile/.4 km up hill; $\frac{1}{2}$ mile/.8 km recovery jog; final section covered in long strides, and ends with a jog back to base.

Hill running
A suitable gradient is needed (footballers make use of the stadium tiers for this purpose). Sprint hard up the hill, then recover and try again. Try 5 runs, building up to 10.

Hopping, jumping, skipping, high kicks, sideways and backwards running are all exercises that will increase leg power and improve stamina, and are particularly important in football training. Although large distances are covered during a football match they are not at an even pace and sudden bursts of energy are required for distances of 5 or 10 yds/4 – 9 m, coupled with longer bursts of 10 to 30 yds/9 – 27 m. To cope with these, training is geared to short sharp bursts aimed at reducing the recovery time and enabling the player to last the full 90 minutes of the match.

Combining these changes of pace with your normal distance running will introduce variety into each outing and provide valuable endurance training.

Translated to everyday life, this training will enable you to cope adequately with life's inevitable stops and starts. You will not pant after racing to catch a bus or after climbing a flight of stairs. Your *recovery* time will have improved; all the discomfort is taken out of short term exertion, and your pulse and breathing return more rapidly to normal.

If you only attempt one form of exercise, then running is the one you should adopt.

56

Fitness and Sport

Getting fit is an end in itself but almost invariably those who become fitter become active in sport (while active sportsmen become fit). And the sense of general wellbeing that accompanies the return to fitness is a powerful stimulus to get out and try a sport of some kind, as an alternative to more sedentary pursuits. Fitness and sport go hand in hand, but while the programmes in this book will make you a healthier, fitter person, able to take part in active sport, all sports activities demand a degree of skill in their performance that can only be learned with practice and repetition. Fortunately there are numerous opportunities to learn about sports and to join sports clubs, and partly because the choice is so wide the following guidelines are offered:

Choose a sport to suit your age
Clearly some sports are more suitable for younger people, as they demand a high degree of fitness and time for training that is probably not available to the older person with the responsibility of a family and a job. This applies to most team sports, including football, hockey, basketball, rugby etc. which will involve joining a club and attending team coaching sessions as well as participating in games. The time taken will be considerable if the level of skill is reasonably high.

Because team games consume a lot of time they attract younger people with fewer ties, so that an older person might find himself out of place in a group of youngsters. This is not to say he should not join if he is fit and skilled enough, but the pace may be above his capabilities and the experience may prove frustrating and disappointing. So do not aim your sights too high and choose an activity that suits your particular age group and responsibilities.

Choose a sport that suits your capabilities
We are not talking simply about skills, which generally can be learned with practice, but about levels of general fitness and body type. Body

57

typing was discussed earlier and we noted how some people are more suited to particular types of activity than others. Accordingly, the tall, rangy ectomorph will tend towards athletics, particularly long distance events, high and long jumps, and team sports such as basketball where extra height is a distinct advantage. The mesomorph is fortunate in being suited to most sports, and can perform well in team games such as football and rugby, as well as in many athletic events. With his considerable bulk and strength, the endomorph is at his best performing feats of strength such as shot putting or weight lifting, but would obviously be at a disadvantage among volleyball players or water skiers.

These are not hard and fast rules but you should attempt a sport that best suits your physical makeup, otherwise you will not perform at your best and will be at a disadvantage.

Choose a sport that suits your circumstances

Team sports demand people, swimming needs water either in a pool or in the sea, tennis requires courts, ice skating requires ice rinks, and so on. So your choice of sport should be guided by where you live and the availability of pitches, courts, pools etc. Fortunately many sports do not require specialised equipment or facilities and even if you live in an area deprived of sports centres, sports such as jogging and running, walking, climbing, camping etc. require little or no special equipment that you cannot provide for yourself.

Some sports are more suited to the country than the town, so that a liking for hill walking and climbing is more easily satisfied if you live out of town, although dedicated enthusiasts will frequently travel many miles at the weekend to take part in the sport of their choice. Do not be put off by lack of facilities provided they do not hamper progress in your chosen sport.

There is also a choice to be made between team or basically solo activities. The former calls for greater organisation and for some facilities, whereas you can walk, run, jog or cycle anywhere you wish at times to suit your own convenience. Budget may also dictate your choice of activity in that, for practical reasons, you may have to opt for fell walking rather than cross-country skiing, canoeing rather than yacht racing.

Remember, however, that the less exotic sports can be just as enjoyable as those requiring large sums of money, and whatever your choice you will find clubs and societies already dedicated to that pursuit and glad to welcome you to their ranks.

In relating your fitness programme to your chosen sport(s), a programme that improves core fitness will be beneficial to all sports activity by improving stamina and all-round strength. Local strength training routines will also help to improve specific performance, for example, the leg exercises undertaken by footballers, tennis players and skiers. However, it is important not to neglect the parts of the body not already worked hard in pursuance of your sport. The footballer, for example, should be concerned about developing his chest and arms, particularly if of slight build, to enable him to withstand the rigours of physical contact that are part of the game. The same applies to cyclists who naturally develop their thighs and lower legs, when chest development will improve their lung capacity and ultimately improve performance.

Many top sportsmen improve the local strength of all parts of the body by using weight in addition to their normal skill training, and their example is one to follow if you intend to progress in your chosen sport.

The Exercises

Warm up – Arms circling

Start with both hands by your side, and your feet comfortably apart for balance (about shoulder width). Bring arms upwards and forwards (1, 2) in a circular motion, back behind your head (3), down and forward again (1, 2).

The arms should brush past your ears and not spread outwards in a 'Y' shape.

Keep up a steady rhythm and repeat about 12 times. Breathe in as your arms go up, breathe out as they come down.

The exercise should then be reversed, arms circling forwards.

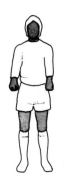

I

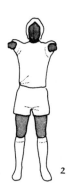

2

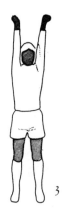

3

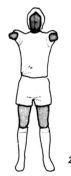

2

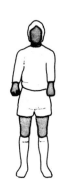

I

*Stand with both hands by your side and legs comfortably apart (slightly more than shoulder width) (1). Bend your trunk to the right (2) reaching down your leg as far as you can. Return to the upright position (1) and repeat 10 times.

Then bend your trunk to the left and repeat the movement 10 times (3). Avoid any tendency to lean the trunk forwards.

** Keep up a steady pace. A variation of this exercise can be performed using a dumbell (5 kg/11 lb) held in one hand. As you reach (4) over to the *right* haul up the dumbell with your *left* hand. As you reach over to the *left* haul up the (5) dumbell with your *right* hand. Note that the dumbell is not used to help you reach further over to the left or right: it is held in the opposite hand to the one reaching down your leg.

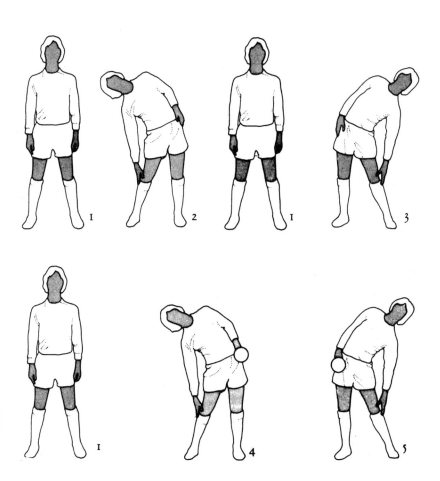

Warm up – Trunk twisting

Start with arms held forward at shoulder height (1) and feet comfortably apart for balance.

Arms are flung to the right, maintained at shoulder height, and the trunk moving from the waist only. The feet stay firmly in position (2).

Maintaining the arms at shoulder height, swing them round to the left (3).

The head should be turned along with the trunk, keeping your eyes on your finger-tips.

Alternatively the exercise can be performed with the hands placed on the hips (4) and maintained in this position while the trunk is rotated to the right (5) and left (6).

10 repetitions should be performed each side.

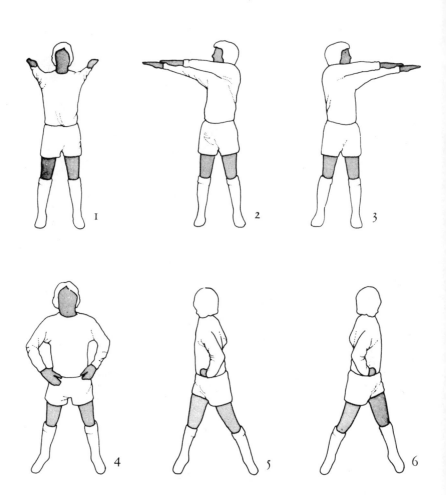

Start with the legs comfortably apart and both arms held aloft (1).

Keeping the legs straight, bend the trunk forward from the waist and touch the right foot with the left hand (2). Return to start position (1). Then bend the trunk forward again from the waist and touch the left foot with the right hand (3).

10 repetitions each side.

* Beginners may not find it possible to touch their toes first time and should aim to reach down the leg as far as possible.

** As fitness improves it should be possible to reach behind the ankle with the hand.

*** Eventually aim to spread the palm of the hand on the floor in front of the foot.

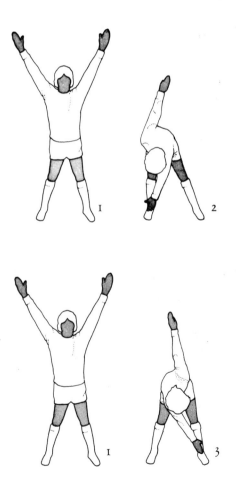

Warm up – Arms flinging sideways

Start with arms held at shoulder height, fingertips touching over the chest and legs comfortably apart (1).

With the right arm maintained in this position, the left arm is flung outwards and extended (2). Return to position (1). The left arm is then maintained in the start position and the right arm flung outwards (3). Return to start position (1) and repeat.

Note that the trunk does not rotate and the legs are held firmly in position. 10 repetitions each side.

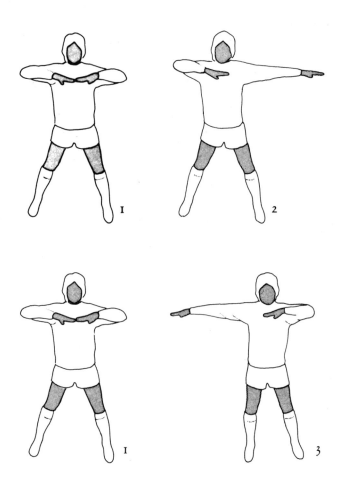

Start in the squat position (1). In a quick movement, palms of the hands are brought face onto the ground and the legs kicked backwards (2) until they reach position (3).

Legs are then brought back sharply (2), to the start position (1).

10 repetitions should be performed at a brisk pace.

** A more advanced method of performing this exercise is shown in figures (4–8).

*** Start in the upright position (4). Throw the body forward (5), at the same time kicking the legs backwards (6/7) reaching the final position (8). Return to the start position (4), by reversing the movement (8–7–6–5–4) and repeat 10 times.

Alternate leg pumps

Note that knee must come up to touch arm and head is held up (9–10).

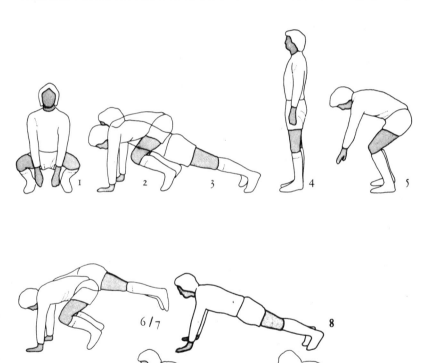

Squat with medicine ball

The start position is shown in figure (1). Body is erect, feet comfortably apart and a medicine ball or sandbag (5 kg/11 lb) held above the head; arms are extended and kept straight throughout.

Lower the trunk to the squat position (2). Breathe in deeply at position (1) and breathe out as you lower the body to position (2).

Return to the start position and repeat 10 times.

*   repeat 10 times
**   repeat 15 times
*** repeat 25 times

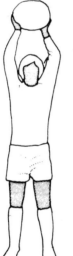

I

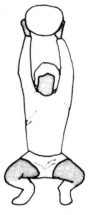

2

Snatch with medicine ball

Start with medicine ball or sandbag placed between the feet, which are comfortably apart for correct balance. Bending the knees, firmly grasp the sandbag (1), and bring it to the chest, at the same time straightening ·the legs (2). Then push above the head (3).
Reverse the sequence and return the sandbag to the ground.

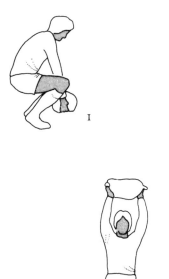

I

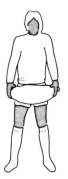

2

3

Skipping

Skipping is an excellent additional warm-up exercise before any serious training session, or it can be used as a substitute for running/jogging, and improves co-ordination and balance.

The standard method is shown in figure (1) ('the boxer's skip') where the exerciser moves lightly on alternate toes.

Variations include the hopping skip, as shown (2) and skipping with both legs together, the knees raised as high as possible (3).

*   1 minute
**   3 minutes
*** 5 minutes

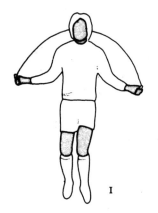

I

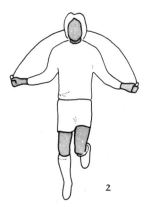

2

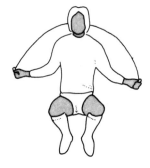

3

*Figures (1, 2) show the easiest form of press-up (or chair dip) suitable for the beginner. Try 10, 15 and 25 repetitions. Note that the back stays straight throughout.

** Figures (3, 4) show the standard push-up. The body again stays rigid and is *lowered* towards the floor. Try not to touch the floor with your body. Push upwards to raise and repeat 10, 15 and 25 times.

*** The advanced push-up is illustrated in figures (5, 6). Feet are raised onto seat of chair (5) and body, held rigid, is lowered to floor ievel (6). Push upwards with arms to position (5) and repeat 10, 15 and 25 times.

All push-ups should be performed at a steady pace and care taken to ensure that the body is pushed upwards and lowered in a controlled movement i.e. do not flop onto the floor. Repetitions are increased as strength is gained.

*   repeat 10 times
**   repeat 15 times
*** repeat 25 times

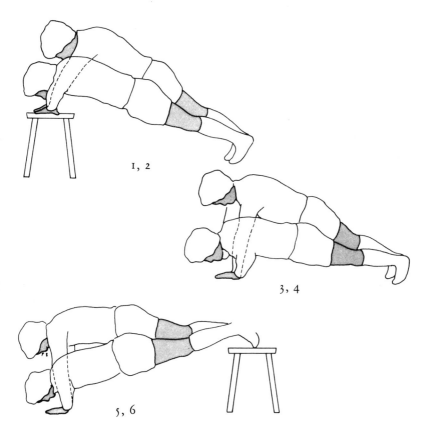

I, 2

3, 4

5, 6

Can be performed with a barbell or dumbell(s).

Figure (1) shows the start position, using a barbell. Feet are set firmly apart for balance, back is straight and arms fully extended. Moving from the elbows only, the lower arm performs a hinge movement (2), raising the barbell to the final position (3). The barbell is then lowered to the start position in a controlled movement and the exercise repeated 10 times.

The weight of the barbell can be increased progressively, starting with a weight you can comfortably manage without straining. The trunk should not be moved to assist the raising of the bar and the bar should not be allowed to 'rest' across the chest. The elbows should remain close to the sides of the body and not pulled in towards the trunk for support.

The same exercise can be performed using a single dumbell or two dumbells (4, 5, 6).

*   repeat 10 times
* *   repeat 15 times
* * * repeat 25 times

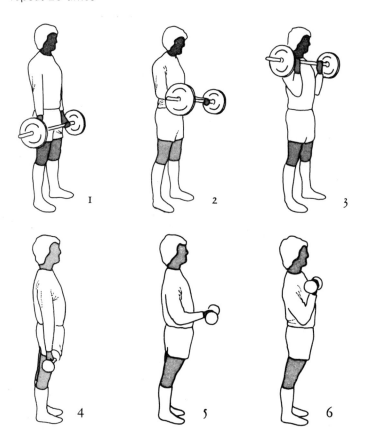

Arms – Dumbell press and alternate dumbell press

Start in position (1) with a dumbell grasped firmly in each hand. Dumbells are pushed upwards until the arms are fully stretched (2). Lower and repeat the movement from position (1).

In the Alternate Dumbell Press, dumbells are raised alternately (3, 4) in a similar movement.

Dumbells are lowered in a controlled movement. Check any tendency for the arms to come forward when in the raised position (2, 3, 4) by forcing them back.

This exercise can also be performed sitting down.

Choose a weight you can comfortably handle to start with, say, around 5 kg/11 lb. Perform 10 repetitions, then increase. Movement should be steady and rhythmical.

*   repeat 10 times
* *   repeat 15 times
* * * repeat 25 times

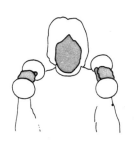

1

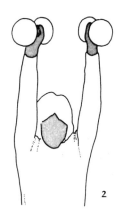

2

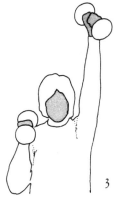

3

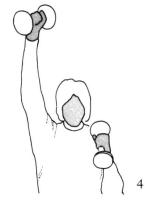

4

Arms — Dumbell lateral raise

A pair of dumbells are grasped and body set in the start position, with legs comfortably apart for correct balance (1). Arms are then raised sideways, up to or slightly above shoulder height (2). Arms are then lowered to start position in a controlled movement. The movement is then repeated.

Repeat 10 times, starting with a weight you can comfortably manage. Weight and number of repetitions can be gradually increased.

A more advanced version of this exercise (bent-over lateral raise) is illustrated in fig. (3). The upper part of the body is bent from the waist until parallel with the floor. The dumbells are then raised upwards and outwards until level with shoulders. They should not be *swung* into this position. Lower gradually and repeat (4).

* repeat 10 times
** repeat 15 lines
*** repeat 25 times

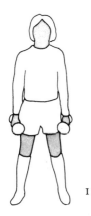

I

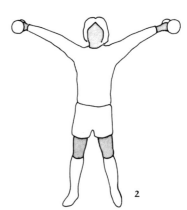

2

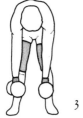

3

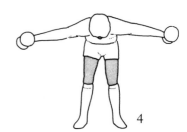

4

A movement specifically designed to exercise the triceps.

A dumbell is held as in position (1), with the arm extended above the head. The arm is then bent from the elbow joint (2), until the lower arm is parallel with the ground.

The dumbell is then raised to the start position (1). All movements should be controlled.

This is a difficult exercise and should be performed correctly. Start with a weight around 5 kg/11 lb and attempt 10 repetitions. Weight and number of repetitions can be gradually increased.

*   repeat 10 times
**   repeat 15 times
*** repeat 25 times

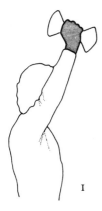

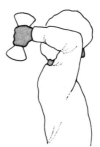

I

2

A useful warm-up/strength exercise for arms and shoulders.

Wooden chair is grasped by its front legs (1) and swung in a full circle (2, 3) over the head. 10 times clockwise, 10 times anti-clockwise.

Note that the arms remain *straight* throughout this exercise.

* *   repeat 10 times
* * * repeat 20 times

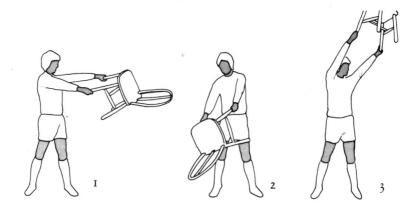

Shoulders – Straight arm lift

A dumbell is held in each hand, arms resting loosely by the side, feet comfortably apart, as in figure (1). The right arm is then raised in front of the body (2) to shoulder height. Hold in this position momentarily and lower to start position (1) in a controlled movement. Repeat the movement with the left arm.

10 repetitions each side should be attempted and dumbell should be around 5 kg/11 lb.

Note that arms stay straight throughout, (3) and the trunk rigid. Avoid any tendency to lean backwards to gain extra leverage.

* repeat 5 times
** repeat 10 times
*** repeat 20 times

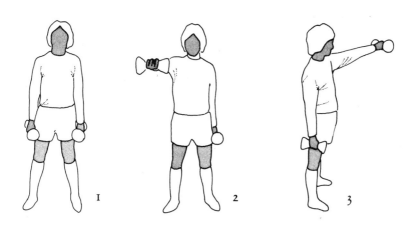

Shoulders – Barbell press behind neck

Start with barbell laid across the shoulders, behind the back, grasped firmly in both hands. Legs are comfortably apart for balance and the trunk rigid (1). Pressing firmly upwards, the arms are stretched raising the barbell to the finish position (2). The barbell is then lowered in a controlled movement to the start position (1) and the exercise repeated.

Try 10 repetitions. Barbell weight 10 kg/22 lb.

Note that the movement is performed by the arms only and any tendency to gain additional thrust by moving the trunk should be avoided. Do not strain the muscles by using too heavy a weight.

*   repeat 10 times
**   repeat 15 times
*** repeat 25 times

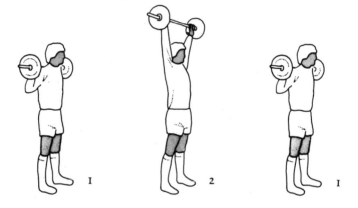

I   2   I

Assume the start position (1), with the hands resting firmly on the seats of two chairs which are set slightly more than shoulder width apart. The body is held rigid.

The exercise consists of lowering the body to position (2) using a controlled movement, and then raising it back to the position (1).

Work at a steady rhythmic pace and attempt 5 repetitions. The number can be increased as fitness improves.

*   repeat 5 times
* *   repeat 10 times
* * * repeat 20 times

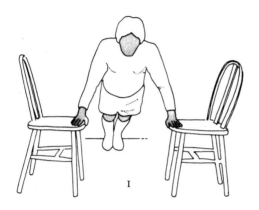

I

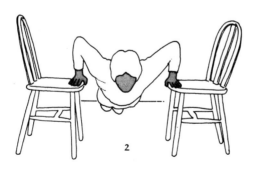

2

A difficult exercise. The trunk is bent forward from the waist with back straight and head up. The arms perform a rowing movement, pulling upwards towards the pectorals.

* At first the exercise should be performed without weights and the emphasis placed on performing the correct movement.

** Then a dumbell of about 5 kg/11 lb weight can be held in each hand and the movement performed.

*** For the Superfit a barbell is used and the exercise consists of pulling the bar upwards and in towards the pectorals. The bar is then lowered in a controlled movement and the exercise repeated. 10 repetitions should be attempted.

Before trying this exercise with a barbell, a broom handle can be used for practice in performing the correct movement.

*   repeat 10 times
**   repeat 15 times
*** repeat 25 times

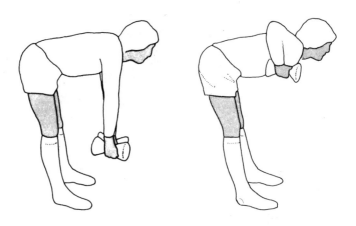

Chest — Chest expansion exercise

Start with arms in position (1), with fingertips barely touching under the chin. Legs are comfortably apart for balance. Maintaining the arms at shoulder height, they are forced back from the shoulders (2, 3) and finally fully extended (4). Return to position (1) and repeat 10 times.

This is a useful warm-up exercise, to be performed before attempting any of the following specialised chest exercises.

*   repeat 10 times
**   repeat 15 times
*** repeat 25 times

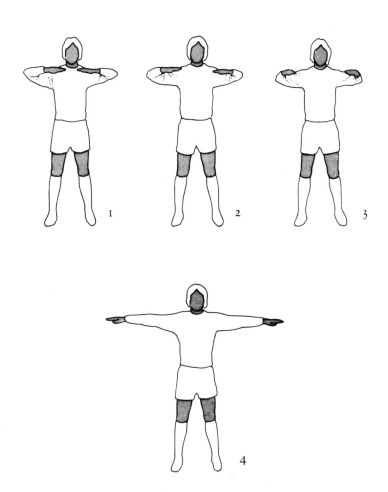

Chest – Bench press with barbell

Lie back on a firm bench (a park bench will suffice) as in figure (1).
Barbell is gripped firmly with both hands, arms are shoulder width apart.
Barbell is then raised to full extent of the arms (2). Lower the barbell to
chest in a controlled movement and repeat. With the arms in this position
special attention is paid to the shoulder/upper arm muscles.

By extending the width of the arms fig. (3) the pectorals are exercised.

Where a heavy weight is used, your partner should hand it to you once
you are comfortably in the start position (1) and remove it from you
on completion of the repetitions.

Try 10 repetitions. Performed at a steady pace, a great stamina builder.
Increase poundage for weight gain and strength.

*   repeat 10 times
**   repeat 15 times
*** repeat 25 times

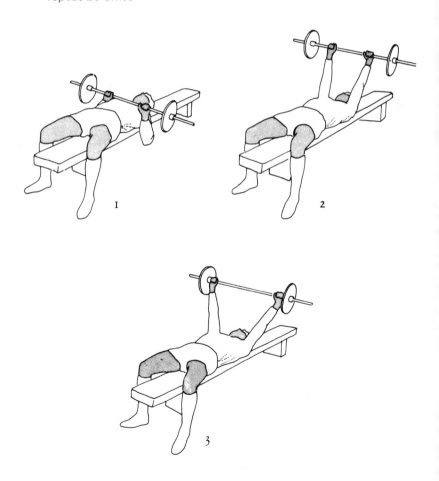

Chest — Expanders or springs

Chest expanders or springs can be used to perform a number of chest expansion exercises. The cables of the apparatus are made either of rubber or coiled metal springs, and the number can be increased as strength is gained.

Figures (1) and (2) show a simple chest expansion exercise. The arms are extended to their full length and the return to the start position is by a controlled movement.

Figure (3) shows a variation of this movement, where the left arm stays still and the right arm only is extended. The positions are then reversed and the movement repeated with the left arm.

Chest expanders or springs can be used to achieve a similar movement to the curl.

One end of the spring is firmly secured beneath the foot.

```
*     repeat 10 times ⎫
**    repeat 15 times ⎬ each exercise
***   repeat 25 times ⎭
```

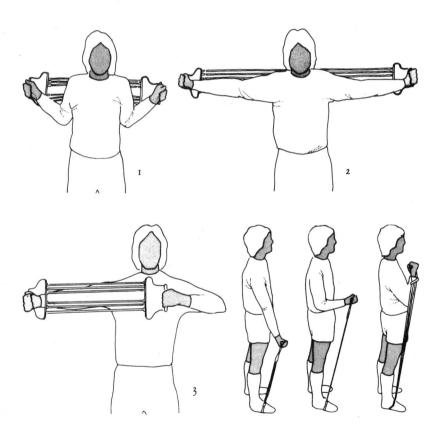

Start position is flat on your back on a bench, with a dumbell held above your chest in each hand. Arms are fully extended (1). In a controlled movement the arms are then lowered sideways, bent slightly at the elbows to position (2). Return slowly to position (1) and repeat. This is a similar exercise to the bench press, except that the arms are allowed to fly outwards in the movement to position (2).

*   repeat 10 times
* *   repeat 15 times
* * * repeat 25 times

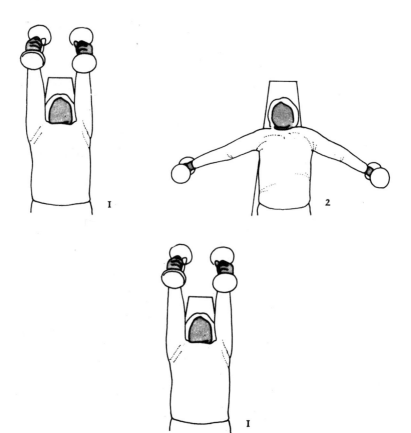

Chest – Straight arm pullover

Lie flat on a bench with a barbell held at arms length over the chest (1).

Keeping the arms perfectly straight, the bar is then lowered behind the head until the arms are fully stretched (or the bar hits the floor) (2). The bar is then raised and returned in a controlled movement to the start position (1).

Note that the hips and legs do not leave the bench/floor.

The exercise can be extended, so that the weight is taken forward to rest on the thighs (3), before returning to positions (1, 2).

*   repeat 5 times
* *   repeat 10 times
* * * repeat 20 times

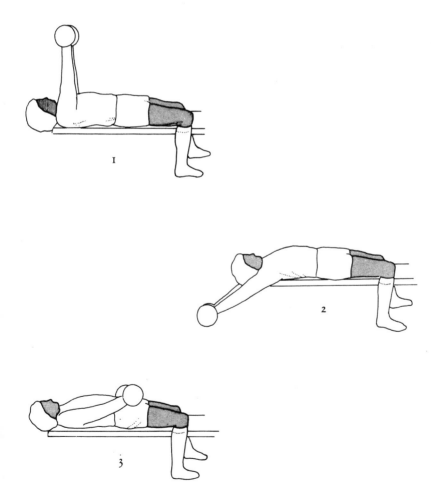

Barbell is held at the hang position across the front of the body, arms fully extended, with the knuckles to the front (1). The hands should be 20 cm/8 in. apart. Bending the elbows, the barbell is then raised to the level of the chin (2). Make sure that the barbell stays close to the body and that the trunk is not bent backwards to gain extra thrust. Lower the bar in a controlled movement and repeat.

*   repeat 10 times
**   repeat 15 times
*** repeat 25 times

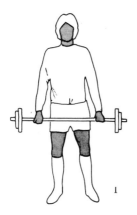

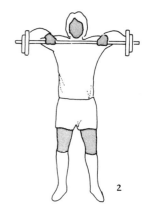

The chinning bar is used to perform a number of movements, where the body is pulled upwards by the arms. The 'bar' itself may be made to fit into a door frame, or you may make use of a convenient tree branch or goalposts outdoors. The basic exercise is to grasp the bar firmly with the fingers pointing away from the body and then raise the body so that the chin is level with the bar (1, 2).

A more advanced exercise is to use the same grip but raise the body so that the bar is behind the neck. This is particularly useful for the back and shoulder muscles (3, 4).

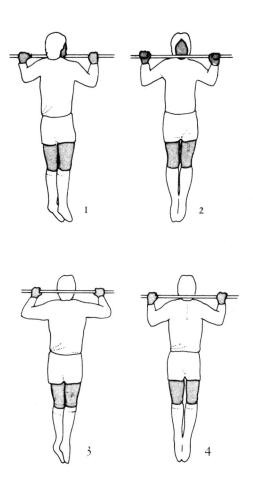

Shoulders – Front (Olympic) press

The barbell is held across the chest, at shoulder height (1). A wide grip is adopted, slightly more than shoulder width.
    The bar is then driven upwards, to full extent of the arms (2). Return in a controlled movement to position (1) and repeat.

*   repeat 10 times
* *   repeat 15 times
* * * repeat 25 times

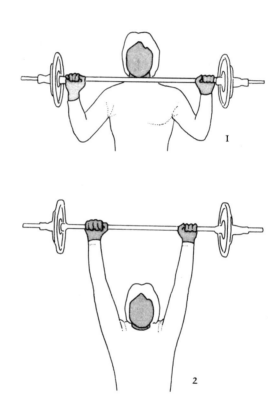

Stomach – Sit-ups

This is a basic stomach strengthening exercise and can be performed in a variety of ways.

Figures (1, 2, 3, 4) show the sit-up on the level, with your partner grasping your ankles to hold them firmly on the ground. Hands are clasped behind the neck as the body is raised. In the final position, the head is forced down towards the knees as far as possible.

The more advanced should be able to perform this movement without the aid of a partner (5, 6). A variation is the twisting sit-up (7), in which the trunk is twisted, so that the right elbow aims to touch the left knee, and vice versa.

A weight (dumbell, medicine ball, sandbag) can be clasped behind the neck to make the sit-up from the level more difficult.

*   repeat 10 times
**   repeat 20 times
*** repeat 30 times

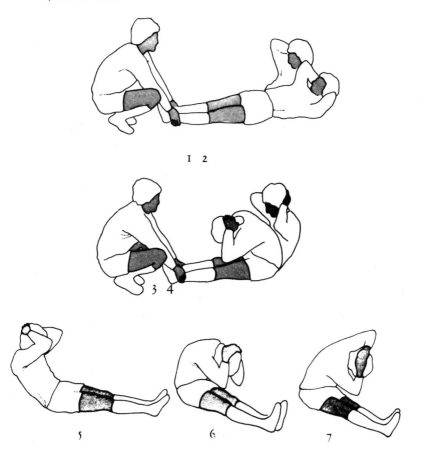

I 2

3 4

5   6   7

More advanced versions of the previous exercises.

The sit-up on the inclined bench can be performed with the aid of a partner and is shown in figures (1, 2). By increasing the angle of the board, the exercise is made more difficult.

Without using a board the inclined sit-up can be performed by placing the feet on the seat of a chair or bench (3, 4) and raising the trunk from the prone position.

Trunk twisting can be performed on the incline, and here your partner's assistance should be sought to hold the feet firmly in position (5).

*   repeat 10 times
* *   repeat 15 times
* * * repeat 25 times

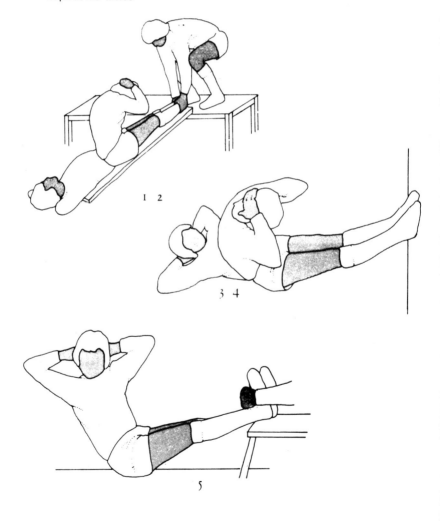

This exercise is performed on a bench, with a partner firmly grasping your ankles. You should sit right at the edge of the bench (1), with hands on hips. The trunk is then lowered from the waist over the edge of the bench (2) in a controlled movement, until position (3) is reached. The trunk is then raised through to the start position (1) and the movement repeated.

** repeat 5 times
*** repeat 15 times

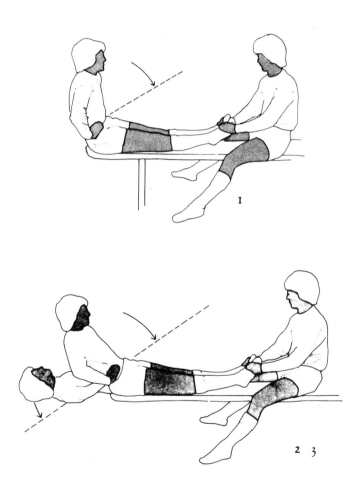

Lower trunk, Stomach and back – Cat stretch – Shoulder bow – Locust

Cat stretch

An exercise aimed at giving mobility to the spinal column.

Start as in position (1), with arms straight. The body is then arched (2) while the arms remain straight. Return to start position (1) and repeat. All movements should be controlled throughout.

Shoulder bow

In this movement the body is arched in a reverse position as shown in figure (3, 4).

Locust

Performed as shown in figures (5, 6). Both legs can be raised simultaneously or alternately. Note that the position of the hands remains alongside the body.

*   repeat 5 times
**   repeat 10 times
*** repeat 15 times

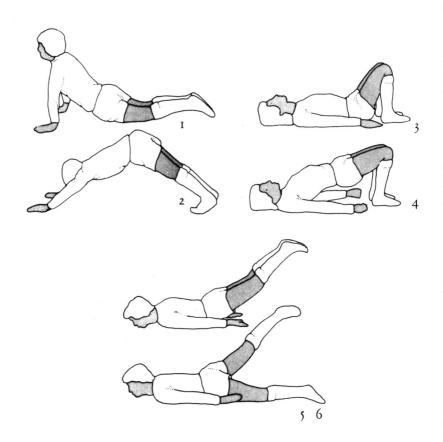

Lower trunk, Stomach and back – Knee bends – Rowing – Back stretch

Alternate knee bending
Assume position (1). The knees are alternately pulled upwards towards the chest and held momentarily.

Rowing
A forward rowing movement is performed (2), with the trunk bending from the waist. Arms are kept straight and made to reach forward towards the feet.

Back stretch
From a sitting position (3), the trunk is bent forwards until the head touches the knees. Arms are used to reach down the legs towards the ankles, which can be grasped to assist in performing this movement.

*   repeat 5 times
**   repeat 10 times
*** repeat 20 times

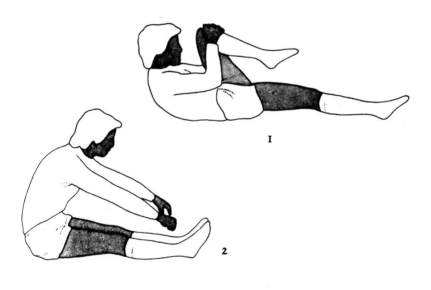

I

2

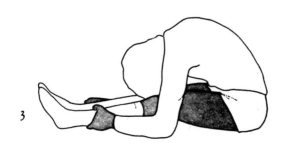

3

From a prone position, arms reach back to grasp the ankles. The position is held momentarily, then released and repeated.

*   repeat 5 times
* *   repeat 10 times
* * * repeat 20 times

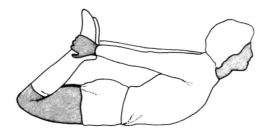

Lower trunk, Stomach and back – Back lift

Assume a prone position, with arms clasped behind the neck and your partner firmly gripping the ankles (1) for support.

The trunk is then raised and forced backwards as far as it can go (2). Lower the trunk in a controlled movement and repeat.

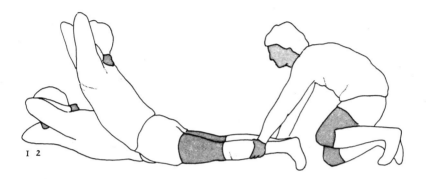

I 2

Assume the start position (1). Note that the legs are straight in the air, the back rigid and the trunk supported by the arms. Bending at the waist the legs are then forced back, until toes touch the floor behind your head (2). Return to start position (1) and repeat.

A more advanced variation is shown in figure (3). Note the altered position of the arms, so that the trunk moves without support. Once the legs are positioned as at (3), a pumping motion is performed, lowering and raising each leg alternately.

*   repeat 5 times
**   repeat 10 times
*** repeat 20 times

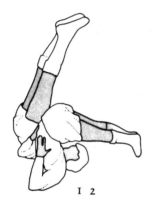

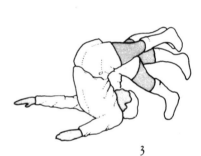

I 2   3

Lower trunk, Stomach and back – Touching alternate toes

From a seated position, with the trunk kept erect from the waist upwards, arms reach out to touch alternate toes (1, 2).

*   repeat 5 times
**   repeat 10 times
*** repeat 20 times

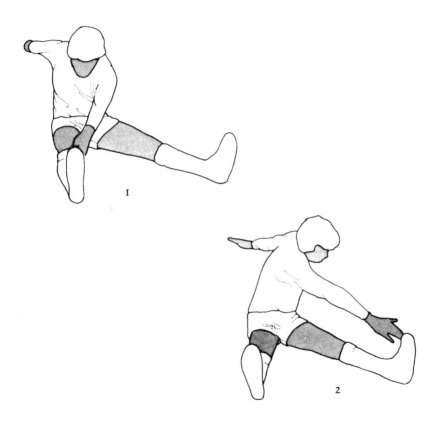

Lower trunk, Stomach and back – Abdomen support

Assume the start position (1), with the stomach resting on a medicine ball. The arms are then raised up and outwards, with the result that the abdomen takes the full weight of the body (2).

In a further movement, the arms can be extended forwards (3).

You should breathe in as arms are raised in both movements.

Return gradually to position (1) and repeat.

*   repeat 5 times
* *   repeat 10 times
* * * repeat 20 times

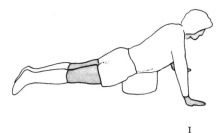

I

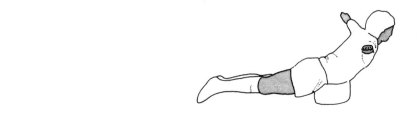

2

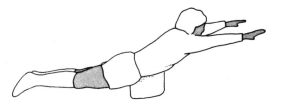

3

This is a basic abdominal strengthener and can be performed with a number of variations.

Start in position (1), flat on your back with arms close to the sides of the trunk. In a controlled movement, legs are raised about 20 cm/8 in. and *held* at this height (2). Open the legs (3), then close, and lower gradually to the ground (do not let the legs drop).

An advanced version of this exercise consists of using a medicine ball or sandbag resting on the shins, while the legs are raised, held and lowered as in the previous movement (4).

*   repeat 5 times
* *   repeat 10 times
* * * repeat 20 times

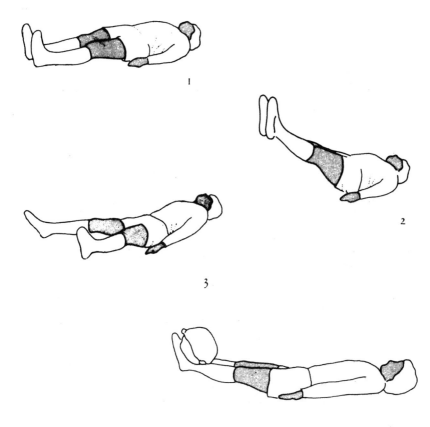

Bicycling
Assuming the position shown (1), the legs perform a bicycling movement in the air.

*   30 secs
**   60 secs
*** 120 secs

Scissors

A scissor motion can be performed in position (2), as the legs are pumped upwards and downwards at a fairly vigorous pace.

*   10 secs
**   20 secs
*** 30 secs

Leg pressure/lift
In this exercise, the left leg is shown pressing upwards, while the right leg (crossed over) is pressing downwards (3). Note that both legs are held at about 20 cm/8 in. from the floor throughout, thus increasing the pull on abdominal muscles.

*   repeat 5 times
**   repeat 10 times
*** repeat 20 times

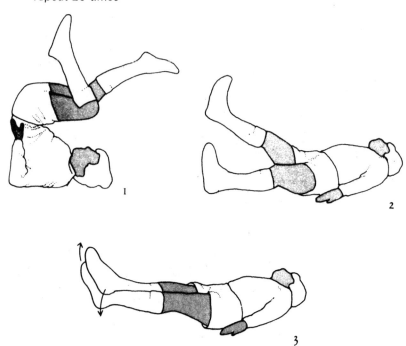

Lower trunk – Legs raise over high object

Assume the start position as shown (1), with the trunk supported by the arms. Legs are then raised to a height sufficient to clear the object (2) and finally lowered in a controlled movement to the ground (3). Use the same movement to return to the start position (1) and repeat.

To start with, a lower height object can be used, such as a medicine ball or the seat of a chair.

*   repeat 5 times
* *   repeat 10 times
* * * repeat 20 times

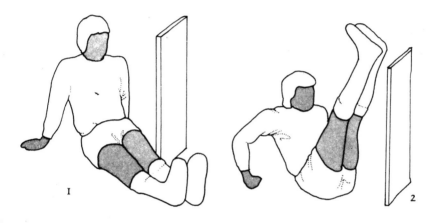

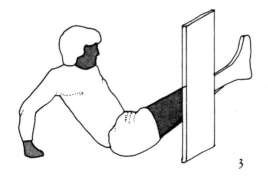

In this exercise the weight of your partner is used as a back/stomach strengthener.

Two partners stand back to back, their arms locked at the elbow (1). The partner performing the lift leans forward (2), raising the second partner off the ground. Hold momentarily and then lower to the start position (1). The movement is then performed by the other partner and repeated (3).

By raising his legs to a right angle with his body, the partner being lifted can use this exercise as an additional stomach muscle strengthener.

*   repeat 5 times
**   repeat 10 times
*** repeat 20 times

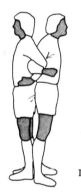

I

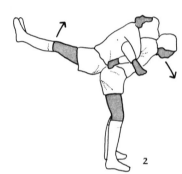

2

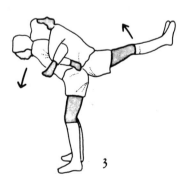

3

Lower trunk, Stomach and back — Squat twist

Assume a squat position, with a broom handle held across the shoulders (1). Keeping the trunk erect — not leaning forward or backwards — the trunk is bent to the right, so that the tip of the broom handle touches the floor (2). Return gradually to position (1) and lean over to the left so that the tip of the broom handle again touches the floor (3). Return to position (1) and repeat.

This exercise will help improve balance and also strengthen the thigh muscles.

*   repeat 5 times
**   repeat 10 times
*** repeat 20 times

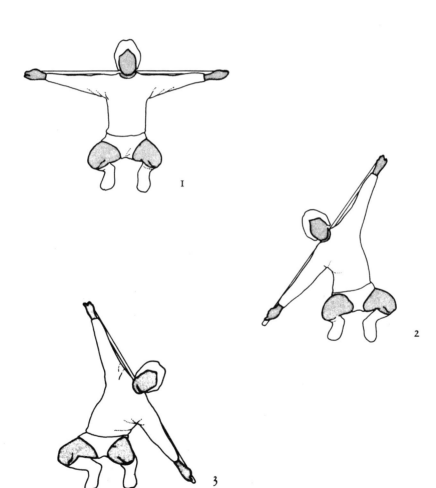

This exercise is particularly useful for stretching and strengthening thigh muscles.

Start in an upright position, hands on hips. Then go downwards and forward on the left leg, bending at the knee, while the right leg stays straight (1). Return to the upright position and repeat.

An advanced method of performing this exercise is shown in figure (2). The 'free' leg is raised – onto a seat, bench or chairback – while the leg being exercised is bent. The trunk is eased as low as possible.

Sideways splits are performed by many footballers before a game and the technique is illustrated in figures (3, 4, 5) where the emphasis is on exercising the groin muscles which are susceptible to strain.

High kicks (6) are another useful loosening/warming-up exercise. Hold one arm outstretched and try to kick it with the leg being exercised.

*   repeat 5 times
* *   repeat 10 times
* * * repeat 20 times

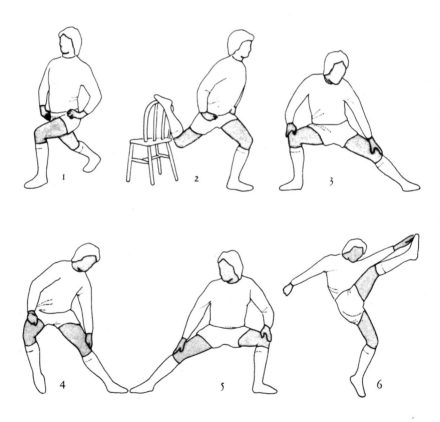

A simple exercise that can be performed using a chair, step, bench etc.

Take up a position in front of the chair (1), and lift the left leg onto the seat (2). Then raise the trunk (3) using the power only of the leg muscles, until the right leg is also on the chair (4). Step down and repeat with each leg.

The exercise can be made more difficult by carrying a weight (e.g. dumbell) in each hand, and for stamina training the pace can be fairly brisk.

A variation of the exercise is to walk up a flight of steps, carrying weights (dumbell, or barbell across shoulders). Walk down again and repeat.

*   repeat 5 times
**   repeat 10 times
*** repeat 20 times

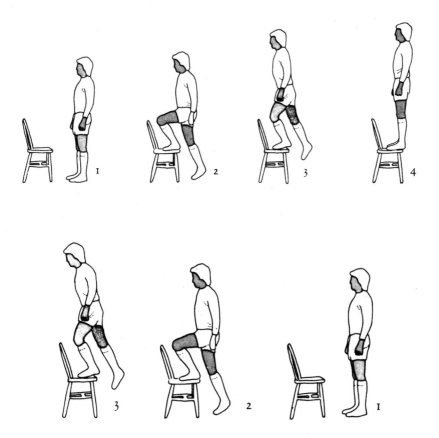

Legs – Squat with barbell

A basic weight training exercise for the thigh muscles.

Barbell is laid across the shoulders (1), feet comfortably apart, body in the upright position. Knees are bent and the trunk lowered (2) until the upper legs are *parallel with the floor* (3), no lower to avoid injury. Raise the trunk to the start position (1) and repeat.

Beginners should practise the squat movement without weights at first, holding the hands on hips.

The return movement to the upright position should be controlled and gradual, not springy or jerky.

*   repeat 5 times
**   repeat 10 times
*** repeat 20 times

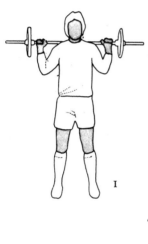

I

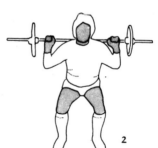

2

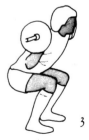

3

Legs – Jumps from squat position

An important exercise for strengthening the thigh muscles and improving stamina.

From the squat position (1), jump into the air as high as possible (2). At this point you can jump into the 'star' shape shown in figure (3), returning to (1).

The same movement can be performed with weights, where a barbell is grasped in each hand (4, 5).

*   repeat 10 times
* *   repeat 15 times
* * * repeat 25 times

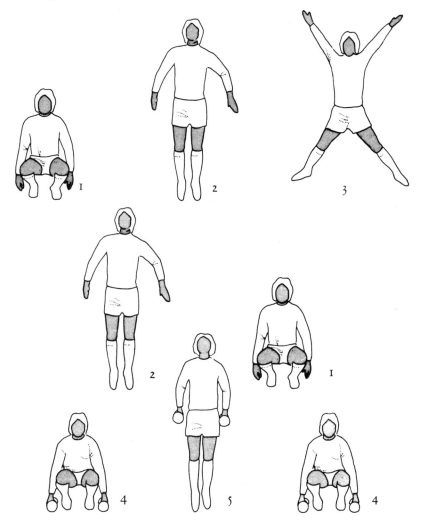

A leg strengthening exercise, using the weight of your partner's body. One partner lies on the ground, arms extended for balance, while second partner lies against feet of the man on the ground (1). The first partner then forces his legs upwards (2) until they are straight (3). Return to the start position in a controlled movement and repeat.

Another useful partner routine is shown in figures (4, 5, 6). One partner lays on the ground, grasping the ankles of the second man who remains standing. First man raises his legs until they are grasped by second partner (4). The exercise consists of the second partner attempting to 'throw' the first man's legs towards the ground (5). The first man tries to resist this movement, using the leg/stomach muscles (6).

Alternatively, the upright partner can remain grasping the legs, while the second man tries to lower them to the ground against resistance.

* repeat 5 times
* * repeat 10 times
* * * repeat 15 times

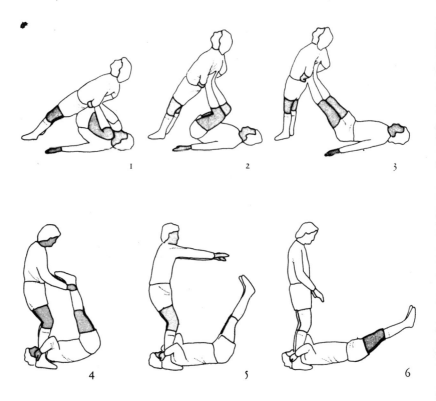

1   2   3

4   5   6

Leg – Toes raise against resistance

An exercise for the muscles at the front of the lower leg.

Partner performing the exercise is seated, with feet firmly planted on the ground and held in place there by second partner (1). Seated partner then tries to raise his feet/toes against resistance (2).

*   repeat 5 times
**   repeat 10 times
***   repeat 20 times

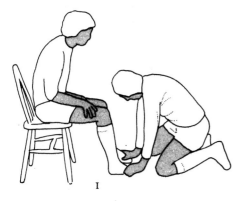

I

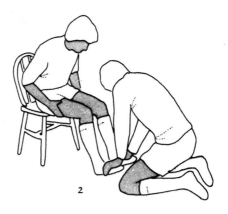

2

The calf muscles (gastrocnemius or gastros) are frequently neglected by sportsmen, and should be exercised by performing a number of movements. These include a number of variations of the Calf Raise.

This movement is performed by standing upright, with the *toes* of the feet resting on a wooden block or shallow step (5cm/2in.) and raising the body in an upward movement. (In the gymnasium a 'calf machine' is used for this exercise; a lever applies weight to the shoulders, and the weight is lifted as the trunk is lifted).

The Donkey Calf Raise can be performed with the assistance of a partner and is illustrated in figure (2).

Rising onto the toes, walking and running on tiptoe will all help to exercise the calf muscles.

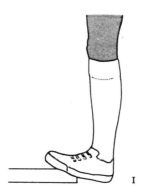

I

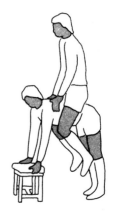

2

Leg – Curl

An exercise to develop the biceps femoris muscles at the back of the thighs and an alternative to using the weight lifter's 'iron boot'.

Exerciser lies prone on the bench with partner firmly gripping ankles as shown. Exerciser tries to draw lower leg towards thighs against the pull of partner.

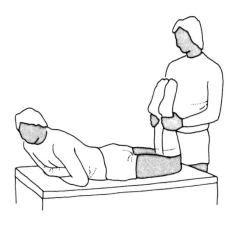

Common Foods: Calories and Nutrients

Beverages	Quantity	Calories	Main Nutrients
Fruit juice	4 fl oz	40/60	Some vitamin C, sugar (if sweetened)
Bitter lemon	1 can	10 per fl oz	
Carrot juice	4 fl oz	20	Some vitamin A
Drinking chocolate, with milk, sugar	1 cup	250	Nutrients of milk, carbohydrates
Cocoa ditto	1 cup	250	Nutrients of milk, carbohydrates
Coffee, black, no sugar	1 cup	Nil	
Coffee, with milk and sugar	1 cup	100	Nutrients of milk, carbohydrates
Colas	1 can	130	Carbohydrates
Tea, with milk and sugar	1 cup	90	Nutrients of milk, carbohydrates from sugar

Alcoholic

Beer	1 pint	180	No food value
Cider	1 pint	300	
Wine, dry	4 fl oz	100	Some minerals
Wine, sweet	4 fl oz	140	
Gin, whisky	2 fl oz	130	

Cheese

Cheddar	2 oz	240	Rich in proteins, vitamin B2, some minerals
Cottage	2 oz	60	Some protein, some vitamin B2
Cream cheese	2 oz	460	Contains fats
Processed	2 oz	210	Contains fats
Cheese spread	2 oz	160	Contains fats

Milk	1 pint	380	Rich in protein, calcium

Cream	½ pint	500	Contains fats, vitamin A
Yoghurt plain	10 fl oz	150	Proteins, fats, calcium and vitamins as in milk
Butter	2 oz	450	Fats, some vitamin B1
Margarine	2 oz	450	Fat, some vitamin A
Eggs boiled, poached	1	90	Rich in vitamin B2, some protein
Fish			
Cod, grilled	4 oz	160	Rich in protein
Fish fingers	6 oz	290	Protein
Sardines, tinned	3 oz	180	Very rich in protein, some minerals
Salmon, tinned	3 oz	120	Some protein, minerals
Meat			
Bacon, grilled	1½ oz	170	Rich in protein, vitamin B1, some minerals
Ham, lean, boiled	4 oz	250	Rich in protein
Beef steak, grilled	4 oz	350	Rich in protein, some minerals
Lamb chop, grilled	4 oz	430	Rich in protein, some fat
Liver, grilled	4 oz	175	Rich in protein, vitamins A, B, iron
Pork chop, grilled	4 oz	550	Rich in protein
Sausages, grilled	4 oz	450	Rich in fats, some minerals
Chicken	4 oz	220	Rich in protein, vitamin B2
Turkey	4 oz	220	Rich in protein
Vegetables			
Beans, runner	4 oz	10	Some minerals
Beans, baked	4 oz	120	Starch, some vitamins
Cabbage, boiled	4 oz	10	Some vitamin C
Cauliflower	4 oz	10	Some vitamin C
Celery, raw	4 oz	10	Carbohydrate (cellulose)
Cucumber	4 oz	10	Carbohydrate, water
Lettuce	1 oz	Nil	Some carbohydrate
Mushrooms, raw, or grilled	4 oz	10	Carbohydrate
Peas, fresh, frozen	4 oz	70	Vitamin B1
Potato, baked	4 oz	100	Carbohydrate
Potato, chips	4 oz	230	Carbohydrate
Potato, crisps	4 oz	650	Carbohydrate
Potato, instant	4 oz	400	Carbohydrate

113

Spinach	4 oz	30	Some vitamins, iron
Sprouts	4 oz	20	Some vitamins
Tomatoes	4 oz	20	Vitamin C

Fruit

Apples	4 oz	40	None particular
Banana	4 oz	80	None particular
Currants, dried	4 oz	300	Some iron
Dates	4 oz	250	Carbohydrate, some minerals
Grapes	4 oz	80	None particular
Grapefruit	½	15	Some vitamin C
Lemon	4 oz	15	None particular
Orange	4 oz	45	Some vitamin C
Peaches, tinned	4 oz	100	None particular
Pineapple, tinned	4 oz	100	None particular
Plums, stewed	4 oz	25	None particular
Prunes, stewed	4 oz	80	None particular
Raisins, dried	4 oz	300	Some iron
Rhubarb	4 oz	Almost nil	None particular
Strawberries	4 oz	28	Some vitamin C
Tangerines	4 oz	60	Some vitamin C

Sweet foods

Sugar, white, brown	4 oz	450	Carbohydrate
Chocolate	4 oz	650	Carbohydrate, some vitamin B1, B2, iron
Jam	4 oz	150	Mainly carbohydrate
Marmalade	4 oz	150	Mainly carbohydrate
Syrup	4 oz	400	Mainly carbohydrate, some iron
Honey	4 oz	330	Mainly carbohydrate
Ice cream	4 oz	230	Mainly carbohydrate, some fats

Bread/flour

Brown	1 slice	70/80	Mainly carbohydrate, some vitamin B, minerals
White	1 slice	70/80	Mainly carbohydrate
Biscuits	1 oz	100/150	Mainly carbohydrate
Cake	1 oz	100/150	Mainly carbohydrate
Cereals (without milk)	1 oz	100	Mainly carbohydrate

Porridge	4 oz	60/80	Mainly carbohydrate (vitamins etc. in milk)

Wheat germ	2 oz	250	Carbohydrate, protein, iron, thiamin, vitamin E

Peanuts	2 oz	330	Rich in protein

1 oz is equivalent to about 28 grams for metric conversion

Diets and Menus

Light/Slimming Diet	Cals.	Moderate to Active	Cals.	Very Active	Cals.
Breakfast					
Fruit juice	60	Fruit juice	60	Cereals, milk, sugar	220
Cereal, milk	190	Bacon and egg	290	Sausages (2), tomato	400
2 slices toast, butter		Toast, butter,		2 slices toast, butter	
and marmalade	320	marmalade	400	and marmalade	320
Tea or coffee	20	Tea or coffee	20	Tea or coffee	20
	590		770		960
Lunch					
Half grapefruit	15	Lamb chop (4 oz)	430	Steak pie (6 oz)	550
Grilled cod (4 oz)	160	Baked beans	120	Chips (4 oz)	270
Peas (4 oz), jacket		Chips (4 oz)	270	Peas (4 oz)	70
potato (4 oz)	170	Ice cream	230	Cheese (2 oz),	
Fruit salad, cream	170			biscuits	350
Black coffee	Nil	Black coffee	Nil	Black coffee	Nil
	515		1050		1240
Supper					
Clear soup, roll	160	Roast chicken (8 oz)	440	Roast beef (4 oz)	300
Grilled steak	350	Salad	20	Yorkshire pudding	130
Chips	150	Roll, butter	250	Mashed potato (4)	400
Salad, no dressing	20	Apple pie, cream	520	Peas	70
Cheese, biscuits	350			Sponge pudding,	
				custard	540
Black coffee	Nil	Black coffee	Nil	Black coffee	Nil
	1030		1230		1440
Daily total	2135		3050		3640

Your Calorie intake depends upon a number of factors – how active a life you lead, your age etc. – but on average a man between the ages of 18 and 35 needs between 2500 and 3000 Calories daily; a growing teenager will require about 3000. If you are very active or seriously underweight, you require more Calories in your daily intake, 3500 or more on average.

By referring to the Calorie guide and consulting the sample menus shown above, it can be seen that whatever Calorie intake you aim for, sufficient variety can be introduced into your meals, and Calories added or taken out of any meal by the simple addition or removal of a course, cutting out roll and butter, going without a sweet and so on.

No allowance has been made for alcoholic drinks or snacks between meals.

Average Ideal Weight

Man (without shoes, clothes)

Height	Small Frame	Medium Frame	Large Frame
5 ft 2 in	108 lb	120 lb	132 lb
5 ft 3 in	111 lb	123 lb	135 lb
5 ft 4 in	113 lb	126 lb	139 lb
5 ft 5 in	117 lb	130 lb	142 lb
5 ft 6 in	120 lb	134 lb	147 lb
5 ft 7 in	124 lb	138 lb	152 lb
5 ft 8 in	128 lb	142 lb	156 lb
5 ft 9 in	131 lb	146 lb	161 lb
5 ft 10 in	135 lb	151 lb	166 lb
5 ft 11 in	140 lb	155 lb	171 lb
6 ft 0 in	144 lb	160 lb	175 lb
6 ft 1 in	148 lb	165 lb	180 lb
6 ft 2 in	152 lb	169 lb	186 lb

Woman (without shoes, clothes)

Height	Small Frame	Medium Frame	Large Frame
4 ft 9 in	89 lb	99 lb	109 lb
4 ft 10 in	92 lb	102 lb	112 lb
4 ft 11 in	95 lb	105 lb	116 lb
5 ft 0 in	97 lb	108 lb	119 lb
5 ft 1 in	100 lb	111 lb	122 lb
5 ft 2 in	103 lb	115 lb	126 lb
5 ft 3 in	106 lb	118 lb	130 lb
5 ft 4 in	110 lb	123 lb	135 lb
5 ft 5 in	114 lb	127 lb	139 lb
5 ft 6 in	117 lb	131 lb	144 lb
5 ft 7 in	121 lb	135 lb	148 lb
5 ft 8 in	125 lb	139 lb	152 lb
5 ft 9 in	128 lb	143 lb	157 lb

Warm-up to Fitness

Six Week Course

Weeks	1	2	3	4	5	6
Arms Circling	10	10	15	15	20	20
Trunk Bending (each side)	5	5	10	10	15	15
Trunk Twisting (each side)	5	5	10	10	15	15
Touch Alternate Toes (each side)	5	5	10	10	15	15
Arms Flinging Sideways (each side)	5	5	10	10	15	15
Simple Squat (support for balance)	5	5	10	10	15	15
Chest Expansion	5	5	10	10	15	15
Cat Stretch	2	2	3	3	5	5
Alternate Knee Bending – Seated (each leg)	3	3	5	5	10	10
Rowing – Seated	3	3	5	5	10	10
Back Stretch	3	3	5	5	10	10
Bicycling (secs)	20	20	25	25	30	30
Skipping (secs)	20	20	40	40	60	60
or						
Running on Spot (mins)	3	3	4	4	5	5
or						
Running Outdoors (miles)	1	1	$1\frac{1}{2}$	$1\frac{1}{2}$	2	2

The above programme is designed to introduce the Unfit person to a programme of exercises and is designed to loosen up muscles and increase mobility. It should last 4 to 6 weeks, before attempting the next stage – Introduction to Strength and Stamina. All routines should be performed at a comfortably brisk pace.

Introduction to Strength and Stamina

	Six Week Course					
Weeks	1	2	3	4	5	6
Berpees	5	5	10	10	15	15
Simple Press-Ups	5	5	10	10		
Standard Press-Ups					10	10
Curls	5	5	10	10	15	15
Sit-Ups	5	5	10	10	15	15
The Bow	2	2	4	4	6	6
Leg Revolve	2	2	4	4	6	6
Abdomen Support	2	2	4	4	6	6
Legs Raise	5	5	10	10	15	15
Splits	5	5	5	10	10	10
High Kicks	5	5	5	10	10	10
Step-Ups (each leg)	5	5	10	10	20	20
Squat with Medicine Ball	5	5	10	10	15	15
Skipping (secs)	60	60	90	90	120	120
or						
Running on Spot (mins)	5	5	7	7	10	10
or						
Running Outdoors (miles)	2	2	$2\frac{1}{2}$	$2\frac{1}{2}$	3	3

Fitness for Life

	Weeks	1	2	3	4	5	6
		Superfit Grades Only					
Press-Ups (Advanced)		10	10	15	15	20	20
Curls'		10	10	15	15	20	20
Press Behind Neck		10	10	15	15	20	20
Bent-over Rowing*		10	10	15	15	20	20
Bench Press with Barbell		10	10	15	15	20	20
Straight Arm Pullover*		10	10	15	15	20	20
Inclined Sit-Ups		10	10	15	15	20	20
Leg Pressure/Lift (each)		5	5	10	10	15	15
Back Lift		10	10	15	15	20	20
Step-Ups (each leg)		10	10	15	15	20	20
Squat with Barbell		10	10	15	15	20	20
Jumps from Squat		10	10	15	15	20	20
Toes Raise Against Resistance (each leg)		5	5	10	10	15	15
Hamstring Exercise		5	5	10	10	15	15
Calf Raise		10	10	15	15	20	20
Skipping (mins)		3	3	5	5	7	7
or							
Running on Spot (mins)		10	10	12	12	15	15
or							
Running Outdoors (miles)		3	3	$3\frac{1}{2}$	$3\frac{1}{2}$	4	4

At the end of each six-week session, poundage of weights should be increased and repetitions revert to week 1 basis until week 6, when further increases can be added with reversion to week 1, and so on. Weight selected should enable exerciser to perform the correct movement at a comfortably brisk pace.

As schedule increases in workload, running – particularly outdoors – can be treated as a separate exercise session to avoid fatigue.

* Special care should be taken to reduce poundage of weight handled for these exercises.

Personal Record Chart

Choose a weight you can comfortably handle for the appropriate exercise.
Increase poundage at the start of each 2 week period.

Weeks	2	4	6	8	10	12	14	16	18	20	22	24	26
Curl													
Dumbell Press													
Dumbell Lateral Raise													
Triceps Extension													
Straight Arm Lift													
Press Behind Neck													
Bent-over Rowing													
Bench Press													
Flyers													
Straight Arm Pullover													
Upright Rowing													
Front Press													
Squats													

Personal
Measurement Chart

Take measurements at start of each 2 week period.

Weeks	2	4	6	8	10	12	14	16	18	20	22	24	26
Weight													
Waist													
Hips													
Biceps													
Thighs													
Calves													
Chest – Normal													
Chest – Expanded													
Pulse – Normal													
Pulse – Peak*													

* Take pulse during middle of run or exercise session before the body has started to 'warm down'.

Index of Exercises